"A wake-up call to anyone who believes that weight management is a quick and easy feat. It's not. And Kuffel's greatest gift is a blast of hopeful reality for any brave reader ready to take herself on and honestly face her own food and weight demons." —Pamela Peeke, author of *Fight Fat After Forty*

"[Kuffel] chronicles nearly every aspect of her life (binges in bed, childhood taunts, depression, meds, sex, breakups, firings, and failings).... It is ultimately and simply Kuffel's own unsparing story that makes [this book] a necessary read." —*Bitch*

"[A book] about women, weight loss, body image, and what we did and did not learn growing up fat, and why losing weight—and keeping it off—is so hard. This is not Valerie Bertinelli in a bikini, promising that if she can do it, you can; this is about 'serial relapsers' and why my cat knows how to eat ice cream off of a spoon. This book is honest, true, and occasionally very funny." —Cheryl Peck, author of *Fat Girls and Lawn Chairs*

"Kuffel's narrative of rededication is a skilled blend of insight ... and emotion ... that never flags in intimacy, honesty, or compassion." —*Publishers Weekly*

Praise for *Passing for Thin*

"Inspiring ... brazenly intimate ... offers a powerful rebuff to anyone who believes that people can't change." —*USA Today*

"[Kuffel's] writing is as clear and sharp as broken glass ... a glorious read." —*The New York Times*

"A talented writer." —*The Boston Globe*

"Empathy, candor, and courage are abundant." —*Entertainment Weekly*

"Rife with snappy anecdotes and mordant humor ... as fascinating in its grotesque insight as in its inspirational uplift." —*The Onion*

"[A] riveting memoir ... grim humor ... A hilarious and insightful book." —*Psychology Today*

Eating Ice Cream with My Dog

*A True Story of Food, Friendship
and Losing Weight ... Again*

Formerly published as ANGRY FAT GIRLS

Frances Kuffel

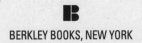

BERKLEY BOOKS, NEW YORK

THE BERKLEY PUBLISHING GROUP
Published by the Penguin Group
Penguin Group (USA) Inc.
375 Hudson Street, New York, New York 10014, USA
Penguin Group (Canada), 90 Eglinton Avenue East, Suite 700, Toronto, Ontario M4P 2Y3, Canada
(a division of Pearson Penguin Canada Inc.)
Penguin Books Ltd., 80 Strand, London WC2R 0RL, England
Penguin Group Ireland, 25 St. Stephen's Green, Dublin 2, Ireland (a division of Penguin Books Ltd.)
Penguin Group (Australia), 250 Camberwell Road, Camberwell, Victoria 3124, Australia
(a division of Pearson Australia Group Pty. Ltd.)
Penguin Books India Pvt. Ltd., 11 Community Centre, Panchsheel Park, New Delhi—110 017, India
Penguin Group (NZ), 67 Apollo Drive, Rosedale, North Shore, 0632, New Zealand
(a division of Pearson New Zealand Ltd.)
Penguin Books (South Africa) (Pty.) Ltd., 24 Sturdee Avenue, Rosebank, Johannesburg 2196,
South Africa

Penguin Books Ltd., Registered Offices: 80 Strand, London WC2R 0RL, England

The publisher does not have any control over and does not assume any responsibility for author or third-party
websites or their content.

EATING ICE CREAM WITH MY DOG, formerly published as *Angry Fat Girls*.

PRINTING HISTORY
Formerly published in hardcover by Berkley Books as *Angry Fat Girls* / January 2010
Berkley trade paperback edition / May 2011

ISBN: 978-0-425-23857-8

The Library of Congress has catalogued the Berkley hardcover edition as follows:

Kuffel, Frances.
    Angry fat girls : 5 women, 500 pounds and a year of losing it—again / Frances Kuffel.—1st ed.
        p.   cm.
    ISBN 978-0-425-23218-7
  1. Obesity in women—Psychological aspects.   2. Compulsive eating.   3. Weight loss—
Psychological aspects.   4. Weight gain—Psychological aspects.   I. Title.
    RC552.O25K84 2010
    616.85'26—dc22

                                                                    2009036037

PRINTED IN THE UNITED STATES OF AMERICA

10   9   8   7   6   5   4   3   2   1

*Penguin is committed to publishing works of quality and integrity. In that spirit, we are proud to offer
this book to our readers; however the story, the experiences, and the words are the author's alone.*

*To Katie, who advised and discussed the issues herein so generously
throughout the writing of the book, and who held my hand
on Saturday nights for a summer.*

*To Lindsay, for calling every morning for a year to prod me
to write, and for pointing me toward the best feminist literature
on the subject of women, food, and weight.*

*To Mimi, whose genius for listening and gentle advice has helped
keep me sane for the last three years.*

*To Wendy, who always called when I was in crisis and kept me
laughing the rest of the time.*

Having loaned me your lives, please accept this portion of mine.

"Then there's only one thing to be done," he said. "We shall have to wait for you to get thin again."

"How long does getting thin take?" asked Pooh anxiously.

"About a week, I should think."

"A week!" said Pooh gloomily. "*What about meals?*"

"I'm afraid no meals," said Christopher Robin, "because of getting thin quicker. But we *will* read to you."

A. A. Milne, *Winnie-the-Pooh*

ACKNOWLEDGMENTS

Most, most loving thanks to my parents, Marie and Leonard Kuffel, for their faith in me, their generosity, their sense of humor, childhood summers at Flathead Lake, and school years full of nuns.

Transcendent thanks to Fredrica Friedman for your faith in me and in this book, and to Denise Silvestro for your passion and your brilliant editing. Andie Avila has been a voice of reason in the editing of a sometimes controversial book and I feel lucky indeed to have had the luxury of two editors.

I'm in debt to Pam Peeke for her brutally tough questions, and to Lybi Ma at *Psychology Today* and Judith Moore at the *San Diego Reader* for encouraging me to delve into this subject before the book was an idea. I wish we'd gotten the chance to be friends, Judith.

Tasha Paley continually kept me in a sense of "we," and Gerry Dempsey and Ann Marie Carley fed me dinner and kept me from reverting to an early hominid when I'd been alone with the dogs and the computer for too long. David Seiter wrenched my heart after I'd given up on men and he keeps reminding me of how lucky I am. Jonathan Elliott's rueful remarks when we meet on the street reminded me I have a brain as well as a useful eating disorder.

My daily peeps—Barley, Boomer, Chance, Henry, Hero, Malachi, and Roger—have owners who have been my cheering section and source of excitement about writing. Thanks not only for the [mostly] Lab Love, but thanks also to

Susan and David Clapp, Ann Allen-Ryan and Leonard Ryan, Susan Sidel, Rene Dittrich and Jo Foster, Grace Yoon and Steve Kilroy, Renette Zimmerly and Tim McLaughlin, and Regina and Steve Rubin for everything you've done for me over the years and for being my most frequent human contact. And if I'm thankful for Lab Love, I have to acknowledge mine, Daisy. She makes me get up and think about something other than myself every day.

I've made forty-two thousand cyberfriends since the beginning of my blogging days. Most of us haven't spoken but you've become a part of my contentment in life.

And finally, but not least, my special love to my brothers, Jim Kuffel and Tom Graves.

AUTHOR'S NOTE

*E*ating Ice Cream with My Dog is the story of finding myself a hundred pounds heavier than when I last committed the crime of memoir. It is also a story of five women, self-named the Angry Fat Girls. This book is based on the spirit of their lives but heavily fictionalized in order to protect anonymity within their families, social circles, and workplaces.

I have created these fictions with their knowledge, active participation, and approval of the book you are about to read. In many ways, they wish they could openly join me in welcoming you to our circle of friendship, but this invitation has been left to me to articulate for them—or me and Daisy, my dog and boon companion, who is asleep with a yogurt mustache on her snout after helping herself to my lunch.

About the Angry Fat Girls

I. After "The End"

In the winter of 2004, I published *Passing for Thin*, an account of my midlife weight loss of 188 pounds and about being part of the world of normal-sized people for the first time. While the critics' response to the book was laudatory, individual reader's opinions ran the gamut from finding me self-involved and heartless to believing me to be a voice speaking about their own body experiences.

I tried and failed to respond to all of the emails. They were painful to read. Many were desperate; some described experiences similar to mine. In the year before the book was published, I began to regain my weight, so I often felt like a liar for giving advice I couldn't follow or sympathy I couldn't give myself. Congratulating the successful either made me twinge with envy or worry that my correspondent would feel my fallibility was theirs.

In the years of regaining half of my weight back, I did not give up on the hopes of permanently resuming abstinence[1] and my 12-step program. I had intermittent periods of abstinence and weight loss. It was during these spells that I was more energetic and buoyant, and I tended to attack my backlog of emails during them.

There have been a number of iconic Poster Girls for Thin in the last several years. Sarah, the Duchess of York, Kirstie Alley, Valerie Bertinelli, Ricki Lake, Marie Osmond, Phylicia Rashad, and Oprah Winfrey have all discussed their weight gains and advocated particular methods for losing. I don't compare my modest fame to theirs, but when it came to my inbox, I, too, found that I'd become a Poster Girl for Thin. But I was a poseur even as the advance publicity for the book began.

II. Frances in Blogland

The genesis of Angry Fat Girls started with the author blog I began on Amazon in the winter of 2006. Initially, I wrote about friendships,

---

1 In food addiction recovery, *abstinence* means refraining from overeating. I'll discuss the various ideologies of this later, but my own abstinence basically means weighed and measured meals, no sugar, and no flour. Fats, protein, and carbohydrates are very carefully apportioned.

dogs, the writing process, having to ask clients for overdue money, what I was making for dinner, why I couldn't fall in love with a man I was seeing. I resolved some loose ends from *Passing for Thin*. I was open about my weight gain and depression, and I came to wonder if I was becoming the Anne Sexton of Amazon.

Mimi—one of the four other women who share the story of *Eating Ice Cream with My Dog*, and the first of the four to comment on my blog—wrote, "I'm glad you are being personal. After reading *Passing for Thin*, I felt as though I'd made a friend who was able to be honest about herself."

I was surprised at how accepting readers were that I hadn't maintained my weight loss. They identified with my seesawing and bingeing. They, too, were between rocky road and a hard place.

"Is there anything else that can make you feel so completely useless and terrible and weak and awful?" B. responded. "It's nice to know I'm not alone in these feelings."

". . . Those of us who feel like freaks for not being able to control a food addiction don't feel like we're the only ones out here . . ." wrote H.

As readers confessed their own stories, ranging from childhood abuse to their diet plans, a string of thanks kept showing up. *Thank you for talking about your weight gain. Thank you for talking about how hard it is to lose a best friend. Thank you for talking about standing up for yourself. Thank you for talking about being depressed.*

By April, my blog became a virtual watercooler in the politics of being female in the new millennium, a place where readers could discuss with each other what they felt other people in their lives didn't understand. "This has become sort of my online diary," M. wrote, and Mimi, one of the Angry Fat Girls you'll get to know, described what was happening most poignantly: "We're all trying to walk new paths without using food as the fix to get there. Working out the kinks, a.k.a. anger, hurt, fear, without feeding them is a process . . . It is like learning how to speak another language. You have to practice it every day."

For women who are afraid to ask for help, the blog functioned as a public red flag in statements rather than pleas. "I'm afraid of airport food, and I came here to get a dose of reality and community," Mimi wrote of being trapped in a late spring Chicago snowstorm.

"I got a lovely lavender dress, and tried it on today after much trepidation, and guess what???? I couldn't get any part of the dress over my HUMONGO upper body!" L. posted.

"I'm sending you a big hug from the west coast," someone wrote back within an hour. "I was a bridesmaid at a size 28 and hated everything about it."

They cheered each other on in successes. "I am impressed that instead of eating, you took the time to stop, take a breath, and write down how you were feeling. It's hard to know what I'm feeling at times."

They consoled each other when they lapsed. "I need to get on here and vent that I gained two pounds at my WW weigh in . . . I *know* that I have not eaten 7,000 extra calories this week," was a familiar lament.

"Hang in there," someone wrote back. "Your attitude is an inspiration that hopefully I can take to heart."

We amassed some hilarious terms for our bodies and food. "I'm stuck with tavern arms," one writer described herself. "I'll save you the gory details of the food porn," a woman said of a late-night brownie session. Wendy, one of the subjects of this book, calls her local deli man the Cheese Pimp. The hang of fat over jeans' tops became known as muffin tops.

Perhaps the greatest compliment to what was happening on my Amazon blog was said not to me, but to one reader from another. "We posted today about the same time (two minutes apart). Our posts are very similar—sugar/chocolate cravings stopped by willpower and reading Frances' blog and [each other's] comments."

Intimacies took place between gardening tips, reading recommendations, parenting ideas, and stories about knee arthroscopy, antidepressants, jewelry, movies, favorite television shows, and housekeeping. Readers became friends among themselves, forming kinships and enmities that I still don't know about. I watched them evolve into a circle of which I was only the Master of Ceremonies.

"I guess I wish I knew what happened after your book, but before these posts. The time in-between. Do you feel like sharing any of this?" D. asked just as my sponsor[2] asked me to write an account of what was then my three-year relapse. I asked my readers if they wanted me to do it in the blog. Their answer was a resounding yes, and for nine days I wrote about what tripped me up and what held me down.

"As I keep stumbling along . . . I keep looking for stories out there of people who battle, perhaps even fall once in a while, but keep pulling themselves up to try again," A. said.

"Please keep telling the story. Been there. This helps," Y. said in confirmation.

The responses turned into discussions of triggers: difficult job experiences, parents, codependency, sugar detox, old habits of smothering our feelings, sugarless candy, lack of time, lack of privacy. Relapse, I learned, was so *easy*, preying on vulnerabilities we ourselves may not know the dangers of. "What precipitated my descent into regaining weight was a despicable act of betrayal by a family member. I was angry at this person, and angry at myself for not making it clear how devastated I was," K. said.

A. confessed, "My birthday fell on a Sunday and I didn't hear from a single friend. Nothing. I spent the day alone. Did some shopping, had dinner out—alone. At the risk of sounding melodramatic, it was the worst day of my life. And I've been on a steady gaining trend ever since."

---

2 In twelve-step programs, individuals seek out "someone who has what you want" to be their mentor, sounding board, last resort. Individuals are expected to be completely honest with their sponsor about their history and current abstinence from the addiction in question.

* * *

I'm going to skip to the end of this book, in March 2007, when the four of us—Lindsay, Mimi, Wendy, and I—who shared the blog Angry Fat Girlz met up in Brooklyn, New York. Lindsay wrote a short post about the experience and among other comments, Belle said, "I would be interested to hear how y'all came to be writing this thing together. I get so much inspiration and thought-provoking insight from your posts and those who comment."

The history of the blog was passed around like a recitation of Homer around a campfire of Athenian soldiers bound for the Peloponnesian battle zones.

L. responded, "Many of Us (capitalized because we thought of ourselves as a club) became regular commentators on [Frances's] blogs, and many of Us came to rely on each other and Frances's insights and inspiration (and her dog stories) for support. Then one day, THUNK! The rug was yanked out from under us and Amazon's blog [mal]function did the yanking. There was no Frances, no Girlz, no support. We finally found each other over on Frances's website, and someone suggested we start a blog. Voilà! Here we are."

"Almost right," Lindsay wrote back. "Wendy started AFG for Frances after the incident she mentioned, and then I came on to help with some of the techie stuff and started posting here and there, and Wendy invited Mimi to join us a little later. We had all been commenting on the Amazon blog regularly. So it's sort of an evolving thing. Wendy is still the official owner of this blog."

Still not quite right, so I corrected: "I don't know that Wendy started it *for* me as much as to provide another platform besides Amazon. I said, 'Sure, why not?' because I'm a blithe soul in cyberspace, but I have to confess I didn't pay much attention to it beyond contributing the name and some of the manifesto. We should ask Wendy why she wanted to start this blog."

As the fire sank into embers, the tale came full around to Wendy. "Why? It just seemed like something to do; some random decision on my part. Sometimes my ideas work, and sometimes they don't. This one seems to be one of the more successful ones."

We decided early on to make this blog more general and issue-oriented rather than a chronicle of our days. We chose to make Angry Fat Girlz a place to discuss popular diet and self-help books, coping with holidays, makeup counters, bra fitting, negotiating visits home, and nights out with friends, Weight Watchers meetings, victimhood, self-sabotage, thin-envy, the Seven Deadly Sins, and cupcakes.

The blog gave women a voice with which to talk about the Great American Pastime that is also the Great American Secret: what we eat, how/when/where we eat, why we eat, how much we weigh, how much we have gained or lost, what size we are, how much we like or hate exercise, the daily aggravations, and the occasional revelation. About twenty readers eventually became bloggers in their own right. Some of those blogs won awards, and some of the writers became new voices for the weight blogging phenomenon.

Of Angry Fat Girlz, P. wrote, "I learned about diet and exercise and Spanx and writing and cooking and shoes and boyfriends and jobs and, along the way, I also learned about personal power."

Wendy, Lindsay, and Mimi had been emailing and hooking up on Instant Messenger while my Amazon blog was most active, forming friendships I had unwittingly instigated but didn't consider myself a part of, although they included me in jokes and articles they emailed each other. One summer night I accidentally turned on Instant Messenger. Mimi found me and invited Lindsay into the conversation. Within minutes, Wendy had appeared online, and I watched them tear apart whatever television show they were all watching. I left my IM open most nights and looked forward to our online conversations-slash-bitch fests. They were hilarious and gave me insights into pop culture that, because I hate TV, I was ignorant of. In June, they had each volunteered to be interviewed for the book on relapse that I was formulating, so I had their addresses from their questionnaires. I sent birthday cards to the summer birthday girls, which meant they then had my address. If I still identified myself with my Amazon blog (and later my blog on Car on the Hill), rather than the Angry Fat Girlz blog, I was enjoying getting to know the women who did the bulk of the work under the initial imprimatur of "a blog for fans of Frances Kuffel." It instantly outgrew me, and Mimi overcame all our laziness at some point and took the tagline off, which was a huge relief.

Out of Angry Fat Girlz, I made three of the closest friends I've ever had.

III. How a Blog Is Not a Book

In March, in the middle of my relapse history, the book proposal I'd worked on for a year was turned down by my editor, and my agent asked what I was writing now. The novel I'd halfheartedly scratched at, I confessed, had taken a backseat to my blog.

"Why are you wasting these lovely, honest entries on a bunch of us reading them here? These would make a great book," J. asked around the time my agent brought up the need for a new book idea. My immediate answer to J. was that, having paid money for *Passing for Thin*, I owed readers my continued candor. By summer, I owed them my gratitude for another book.

The sympathy and stories of my readers' own relapses, I told my agent, assured me that relapse was a topic that was common and little talked about.

I didn't want to write a book based on the blog. Certainly, there would be wonderful information there to use as diving boards for deeper reflection and I'd use bits of it for color, but a blog-book could only be organized in two ways: chronologically or thematically. There was nothing chronological about the blog except the dates of the entries, and nothing thematic except for snippets of back-and-forth over yoga or peonies or fat caste systems. These online dialogues usually petered out in a day or two.

But maybe, I said to my agent, the subject of relapse could be a book, based on more voices and experiences than my own in exploring the special shames of relapse.

I asked if readers would be interested in telling me their stories and my inbox overflowed. Their generosity was partly in support of my enterprise and partly therapy for them as they aired secrets to someone they knew understood and would not be dismayed. The interviews were long and draining on both sides.

The fourth Angry Fat Girl I came to love and share my life with was Katie. Katie can be an over-the-top online contributor or, for reasons that include fear and a doomed sense of distance from the world, a lurker. She did not participate as a commenter on either Amazon or Angry Fat Girlz but she volunteered to give me her weight history. Our connection was instantaneous.

What did I want this book about regaining weight to say? I thought about Andrew Solomon's *The Noonday Demon*, and I thought about its subtitle: *An Atlas of Depression*. I wanted to map relapse and how, more ashamed than ever, we fight back.

I recently received an email from a reader who wants to be an opera singer and is losing weight toward that goal. Our reasons for that first big weight loss have different specific motivations, but in essence they are all about being able to do things we can't do, or think we can't do, when we're fat. Being newly thin after a long/permanent sojourn in obesity is also experientially similar. Compliments, acceptance, no shame at the doctor's office! Clothes! Dating! Climbing, dancing, cycling, the revolved half-moon yoga pose! Maui! Graduate school, career change! While all these exclamation points are deserved, the rewards of being thin have less to do with becoming a superwoman than they do with having the same choices everybody else has.

The illusions have worn off when we are coming out of relapse. Those glamorous mysteries are no longer there. Perhaps the ambition of losing that big weight again is vital to our definitions of ourselves and our bodies because we are forced to assess reality. Mimi, for instance, is no longer interested in weighing 140 pounds, the upper end of her medically ordained ideal weight. She would like to settle at 180 for the sake of her knees and sleep apnea, comfort on planes and finding clothes. On the other hand, I want to get back to 150 for a smattering of venial reasons. I found power in being a size 6, although it was incomplete and I didn't know how to use it. For the first time in my life, for whole minutes at a stretch, I felt unassailable.

Regaining weight is natural and, statistically, nearly inevitable. Being prone to obesity is a physical condition like epilepsy or asthma—at best controllable but never curable.

And yet the participants in my blog kept trying to lose and/or maintain weight, just as forty-five million other Americans try each year, dreaming of one or more of the promises of being thin—professional success, romance, clothes, looking normal, approval from loved ones, improved health and mobility.[3] However, it is especially painful for me and others like me who took years to lose more than one normal body weight and went through the initiation into normalcy only to lose our way and relapse with significant weight gain. I had maintained a weight of 150 pounds for a year. Why did I and so many other women react to life events by savaging ourselves?

I wanted to answer this question, and I wanted to find my way back to being thin. Could I lose my regained weight and invite readers to come along for the ride, either as witnesses or as participants? And if I couldn't lose the hundred pounds I'd put on, perhaps I could document why it's so hard as an offering of reassurance that, no, my readers are not the only ones to regain and get stuck.

---

3   Christine Lagorio, "Diet Plan Success Tough to Weigh," CBS, January 3, 2005.

* * *

Two comments have stuck with me every day since 2006.

The first was an enraged troublemaker, those responders that are called "trolls" in cyberspeak. "If y'all are so over your anger or working through it and well on the way to being 'forgiving' people (whatever that means), then how come y'all are still stuffing your faces with food guaranteed to wreck your bodies? Where, exactly, does that impulse to self-destruction come from, hmm?"

E. responded directly to what was behind that snottiness. "Sharing is HARD. You bare your soul and hope that someone connects. And here, usually they do."

But, despite support and therapy, drugs and journaling, self-help books and exercise, why *were* we all stuffing our faces?

The second comment was harder to absorb, partly because I cried so hard when I read it. "I wouldn't be alive today if Frances Kuffel hadn't gained weight back."

That might be the moment I had to reconsider my weight gain as a positive crisis. *Passing for Thin* included an apt description of life in a fat body, but as I lost weight in the book, it may have become an arrow to the heart of those who couldn't cross the line into a normal size. Poster Girls can be motivators, but they can also be accusers.

In *Passing for Thin*, I tried to tell readers that if I could lose weight, anyone could. However, my blog took on a new mission of putting words to the feelings of failure and shame of regaining weight or being unable to lose it, and of getting on with life as I carried that knowledge. The responses showed how much women needed to speak out about their day-to-day struggles with food and their bodies in the context of their lives, and that they needed each other to understand and share their struggles. I have that in my twelve-step program, but it's a luxury only those desperate enough to dedicate themselves to such an endeavor get. While many of the commercial diets include counseling sessions along with weigh-ins, online bulletin boards, and discussion threads, what I saw in my blog was different. Such venues don't parse the minutia of negotiating life—a toddler's meltdown, panic over a dissertation proposal, or an episode concerning sizism on *Boston Legal*—as *part* of negotiating our relationships with our food and our bodies.

I've never advocated that a twelve-step program is the only way to lose weight, leaving my recommendations to "whatever works for you." But I've discovered that this Weight Thing is clearly easier to bear within a system of sisters. That I, the most meager of icons, had fat feet of clay provided permission for other women to stand up with the safety of anonymity and say, "Me, too," and then go on to say a whole lot more.

One of the questions writing this book has forced me to confront bluntly is where, exactly, does my responsibility for my weight lie? Am I exonerated because of biology, the pain of my history, and/or my dysthymic depression? Or will losing weight contribute to the remission of those conditions?

In the name of all the women I've spoken to or heard from, the broadest answer I can find is that the first steps in taking responsibility are to *name* the problem and then *own* it. The blog world was a chance to own and share our weight problems. Even if we stayed in the ownership stage too long, each of us was more conscious than ever before of what we as individuals needed to do next. I read as women went into therapy for the first time, signed up for their first marathon, left smothering marriages, went on hospital Medifasts, had gastric bypass, joined twelve-step programs, went on antidepressants, got pets, went back to school. Those choices were the next step in the maze of losing and sustaining weight loss.

Another subject this book has prompted me to examine closely is what authentic life is and how it relates to what we weigh and what we eat. *Authenticity* is popularly defined as living by one's core values, which should produce a sense of being at ease with the world and one's missions in life. Aspects of authenticity include:

- Being open to experience without censorship or distortion
- Living fully in the moment, so the self feels fluid rather than static
- Trusting inner experience to guide behavior
- Feeling free to respond rather than automatically react to life events
- Taking a creative approach to living, rather than relying on routine and habit.[4]

Using fat and what I call wrong-eating as a barrier to the outside world impinges on these characteristics. And yet fat women and compulsive wrong-eaters have accomplished great things. The question of authenticity splits at this point. Is genius exempt? Did Gertrude Stein fail herself, or would she have been more if she had been less? Or did being fat and overindulging shape her ability to live without regard to social norms but in compliance with her own creative instincts?

The desire to be at peace with ourselves and the world is not unique to the women who fall into the category of Angry Fat Girlz, but it is a more agonizing search because there are more extremely difficult hurdles of different sorts to overcome. Do doughnuts prevent me from hearing the truths going on around me? Are these fifty pounds keeping me from trying a master swim class? Are these fifty pounds why I didn't get the ER nursing job I interviewed for?

And, conversely, does the search for authenticity we hope dieting will further intervene in living fully? Will my commitment to weight loss continue to isolate me, now in new ways? Can I survive the family reunion with all those desserts around or should I cancel? Have

---

4   Karen Wright, "Authentic and Eudaimonic: How to Go with Your Gut and Be True to Yourself," *Psychology Today*, May/June 2008.

I missed seeing a neighbor because I was looking at the reflection of my new figure in a car window? The what/how/why we eat and what we weigh can be broken into a million Freudian interpretations and causes, but they combine into two fuels that combust when they meet—denial and shame. Double the shame when the woman has relapsed and regained weight, and don't try to quantify the anger. I lied through my wistful teeth when I defined the Angry Fat Girlz blog manifesto as being, "We're not angry at a world that doesn't like fat people, or angry at ourselves. We're angry at our fat, our eating, our reasons for eating." I wanted my weight-and-binge worrying comrades to forgive themselves, certainly. We are all working against biology in the endeavor to control our mouths and pounds, but my anger at what prompts me to eat and at allowing it to get the upper hand was a screed written across the 250 pounds I weighed in March 2006. And despite having a lover at the time and piles of Fat Lady catalogs with nice clothes and open credit lines, I was angry that pretty, feminine, sexual, wantable started somewhere under size 18. I was even angrier at not knowing if that social standard was an external or internal pressure, although I had evidence and a therapist that suggested I put those adjectives aside.

I leave it to my readers to decide these matters of responsibility, authenticity, anger, self-denial, rejection, and girliness for themselves. In *Eating Ice Cream with My Dog* I can only speak for myself and the four women I got to know so well that they share the story of a year of trying to dig out of relapse with me.

IV. The Truth about the Angry Fat Girls

Truths are complicated because truth is both an ideal and an idea, the latter of which has confounded humankind through 2,400 years of debate from Socrates to Pope Benedict XVI. The definition of truth includes conformity to fact and fidelity to a standard. The word derives from the Old English *trēowth*," which connotes loyalty, honesty, and good faith. But history has proven that truth is malleable, and it only takes a reexamination of an issue such as the Jim Crow laws to see how easily truth changes—and loses—meaning.

A *fact* is "information presented as objectively real," and it derives from the Latin *factum*, meaning a deed or an act. A fact is a single thing. The standards against which it is held make up the fluid truth.

In my love for and sometimes frustration with my friends, I have written and interpreted with *trēowth* but I also relied on *verisimilitude*, which is the appearance of truth. The characters Mimi, Wendy, Katie, and Lindsay are based on real people—my dear friends—but are an amalgam of facts and informed guesswork on my part and on theirs about each other's thoughts and motivations. To protect their privacy, I have changed their names, the names of the people in their lives, and their specific locations. I also changed their professions and interests, instead creating fictions that are parallel to their real lives and reflect their truths. I have done this in close consultation with them, constantly asking, "Does this feel right?" One of the Girls has actually taken up the fictional corollary I created for her as a real-life undertaking.

As a memoirist who stuck to the bones of facts in my first book, I know that facts accumulate more facts, like dog hair or a good fit of the giggles, always *growing*, always piling up. I have a healthy distrust of facts because of this messiness, because they give way to new facts and, therefore, become moving targets of truth, which are still always there, in the background, as static, haunting, and untrue as your sixth-grade crush's name inscribed in cement.

If I have had to bargain truth against facts in the pact I made in exchange for the privilege of complete access to four women's lives, I have written about myself in the primary definition of truth, in conformity to fact, except for changing some names.

I have not changed the weight histories, relationship status, and ages of Katie, Lindsay, Mimi, Wendy, or myself. Here are some facts from March 2006:

Frances Kuffel: Fifty years old, five feet eight inches, ever single
Current weight: 250 pounds, size 24
Lowest weight as an adult, at age forty-seven: 148 pounds, size 6–8
Maintained for fourteen months
Top weight, at age forty-two: 332 pounds, size 32
Pounds to lose: 100

Katie Monhan: Forty years old, five feet six inches, divorced
Current weight: 427 pounds, size 5X
Lowest weight as an adult, at age thirty-seven: 140 pounds, size 8
Maintained for one year
Top weight, at age forty: 427 pounds, size 5X
Pounds to lose: 262

Lindsay Longhetti: Thirty-five years old, five feet seven inches, married with no children
Current weight: 172 pounds, size 12–14
Lowest weight as an adult, at age twenty: 132, size 8–10
Maintained for three years
Top weight, at age twenty-nine: 220 pounds, size 16–18
Pounds to lose: 16

Mimi Barth: Fifty-two years old, five feet three inches, ever single
Current weight: 260 pounds, size 22–24
Lowest adult weight, at age twenty-three: 145 pounds, size 14
Maintained for three months
Top weight, at age forty-six: 340 pounds, size 5X
Pounds to lose: 80

Wendy Wicks: forty-seven years old, five feet nine inches, separated but not divorced
Current weight: 270 pounds, size 20–22
Lowest adult weight, at age twenty-nine: 198 pounds, size 16–18
Maintained for two years
Top weight, at age forty-five: 339, size 26–28
Pounds to lose: 90

Total combined weight-loss goal in pounds: 548

Here is some additional information you can carry into reading this book.

Katie is, in a word, nuts, which made for difficult conversations. There is some inability in her to narrate in a straight line and, a native Californian who speed-talks like a Brooklyn lawyer, she relies on how things *feel*. Finding out what those things were or when they happened was like pulling teeth. I think she assumed I knew more about her than I did. Writing this book has involved more phone calls to get Katie's time line right than with any other interviewee.

There's a twelve-step adage that fits Katie perfectly: When a non-addict gets a flat tire, she calls AAA, but when an addict gets a flat tire, she calls 911. Katie is the crisis queen of the book, and sometimes every movement, every encounter, every thought was a physical and emotion hurdle that she had to be coached through.

In Katie's world, there were few people on her side and no one who understood her for long. These feelings proved themselves to be both true and untrue, but she always waited for a friend to become an enemy and for insensitivity to show itself. Her story isn't tangled into the friendships that developed between Lindsay, Mimi, and Wendy because she distrusts klatches in which it's too easy to form sides. She knew that I viscerally understood her physical condition, and she trusted me for my brutal self-revelations in print and in cyberspace; I understood that Katie was someone in need of the pampering that a lot of fat women don't get and cheerleading that, partly through her tense wait for disappointment, was missing in her life.

Katie was the most childlike of the five Angry Fat Girls, unable to wait to open a present on Christmas or her birthday, demanding to know what someone thought of the present she sent. She loved kids and doing kid things like going to the zoo. Our senses of humor were most alike, and we turn sarcastic and gritty when we talk to each other. Almost from the start we adopted a nasal drone in greeting each other. I always knew it was Katie calling when I heard the drawn-out, shallow vowels of my name: "Fraaann—cesss . . ."

Katie is as Irish as the Hills of Tara, although she wishes that she came from a Brooklyn Jewish family. She has auburn hair and sparkling green eyes, freckles and a big smile. At her highest weights, as was true for all of us, her face was dwarfed by her body, but she was lucky in that her eyes had never been swallowed up in fat, although they appear big when she's thin—as does her nose. Thin isn't always fair.

Wendy was the most eager to be interviewed, and she was the one case of hero worship among the Angry Fat Girls, an attitude that embarrasses me (I'd failed, after all), scares me (I am *not* Jesus, the Oracle of Delphi, and Sigmund Freud rolled into one person), and sometimes makes me distrustful (I have no star for you to hitch your wagon to). Interviews were difficult both because she's hard of hearing and because she had a hardcore, deep-woods Virginia accent. Her words could get mangled between these two facts, and her voice often sounded like the unfortunate cliché of fingernails on a blackboard. Writing was often her preferred métier but she tended to get wrapped up in her sense of humor, which I didn't always share. But I have laughed genuinely at her writing when it's about her quirky history. The question she posed to her father about whether she'd ever eaten possum or the fight she had with her mother about her messy car in the church parking lot: this was Wendy at her most authentic.

Wendy is the most socially driven of the five of us. We met during her protracted separation from her husband when she was desperate to find a boyfriend. A prodigious reader, music buff, TV and movie watcher, Wendy subscribes to the *New Yorker*, is obsessed with Queen Victoria, and haunts the National Gallery of Art whenever she gets up to Washington, D.C. My first poetry teacher, Richard Hugo, called such people "culture vultures," and it means that their drive is more class- and in-crowd-driven than it is thirsty curiosity. As a culture vulture, Wendy is the least introspective of the Angry Fat Girls. Her bouts of distress, I learned, often started off about one thing only to morph into another as I pressed further into what was bothering her. She might call in tears over a conversation with her boss when it was seeing her ex-boyfriend's girlfriend the day before that was at the root of her wailing. When the AFGs suggested that she needed to fill the hole he left in her life, she would talk about online dating or harder workouts at the gym to lose more weight. It didn't occur to her that taking a class or finding a church or taking bridge lessons—i.e., not filling the ex-boyfriend hole by finding another boyfriend who's really meant to make the ex-boyfriend jealous—was a permanent way of filling a hole.

Wendy is the only Angry Fat Girl who has never been thin in her adult life. Among the many and complicated feelings I have for her is a physical retraction in her presence, and this demonstrates how well I lie to myself. I'm five feet eight inches, not a shrimp, but Wendy is a couple of inches taller and she seems so *big* despite our being closest in clothing size among the AFGs. She is rawboned and lantern-jawed, and she has a long stride and keeps her head down when she walks as though her destination was clear and near, giving a sense of hurry that takes up yet more metaphorical room.

Her favorite thing about herself is her red hair. She is prettiest when she is grinning; it softens her face.

As the instigator of Angry Fat Girlz and a compulsive reader of other blogs, Wendy had the scoop on what the respondents' real names were on Amazon and on our shared blog, what each did for a living, if they were married, if they were happily married, what method they were using to lose weight, and how well it was working. Every holiday merited a card, every bout of blues was a summons to leave her desk and call the person in crisis, every item of clothing that became too big was passed on to someone a size beyond her. She was and is underemployed and bored, generous and sympathetic, eager to learn and devoid of the innate talent for self-study, and starving for love. Such a personality could be dazzling and overwhelming.

I loved Mimi from the start. She is fact oriented and pragmatic. Her email signature never varied: "Sometimes men are just stupid," and it was a philosophy for her rather than an accusation. It meant, "Pull yourself together. Learn to stand on your own two feet. Depend on no one for free help or sympathy. Trust your own kind."

Mimi is irreproachable. That was her ironic summary of what it meant to be the oldest child and a girl in her family. "You're right, I guess," I conceded to her admonition that I couldn't afford to bid on a mink coat on eBay.

"Of course I am," she chirped in her smug Mary Poppins voice that is saved by a combination of irony and girlishness. "I'm perfect."

Also part of being the oldest was how hard she worked in one profession, making her the most tenured and stable of the five of us. She has moved around all her life, living in Tennessee, Texas, North Carolina, Pennsylvania, Vermont, and while she has some close professional friends, she has few personal friends, preferring her own company so that she can cook, garden, work on her blogs and website, and pursue her many interests. Mimi and I get excited about Chinatown and the Qi Gong massage joint on Grant Street, share a love of Christmas festivities, and have similar tastes in movies. I consider her my closest all-round friend. There are friends who might know me better, but they weren't present for me in the way that Mimi was—my best friend from first grade and I rarely touch base, for example, and B.J. is my best bud on the streets of Brooklyn Heights but is mercurial and prone to grudges. Yet Mimi, who probably has fewer friends than I, would not say the same of me.

Mimi is the prettiest of the AFGs. She has the looks of a Victorian German doll—a lustrous, porcelain complexion, blonde hair, blue eyes, and a pensive sweetness. She has a sexy voice, smooth as maple syrup, girlish, but backed up by intelligence and confidence.

I liked and admired Lindsay from our first conversation. She is a perpetual student, simultaneously seeing herself as a slacker and the lifeblood of practicality in her marriage and in her Italian family. She was working on a doctorate during the time I wrote this book and was an invaluable resource for literary theory and a support via the daily early morning phone calls we made while working on our writing commitments. Lindsay was the most cautious interviewee I had. She, like Mimi, is an old soul. It is hard to remember that she is nearly twenty years my junior. She is fresh-faced and wears her dark hair long and straight, owning the prerogative of a jock and graduate student's exemption from primping.

Despite her managerial talents, Lindsay has a streak of naïveté, partly because of her age. She had been to her grandmother's hometown in Italy and to Boston when we started Angry Fat Girlz, but had lived in Ohio her entire life and married straight out of college. There was an apparent safety net as she dabbled around trying to figure out what to do with her English degree. When I compared her to us other Girls, I didn't have the same sense of walking a tightrope with little training for the stunt. Was it because her weight had never achieved superobesity? Was it because her family was near at hand? Or was it that, in a crisis, Lindsay's practicality and self-protection take over? There is little spillage when she is in duress and she looks doggedly for answers to painful problems. Joining the Spiritualist Church may not appear to be a practical way to mend a marriage that is in trouble and yet Lindsay found a deep sense of connection there that helped give her the strength to seek out remedies for the specific problems she and her husband faced.

Over time, I saw us assuming roles in our small circle. Mimi's empathy and genius for listening gave her the role of a mother, while

Katie, with whom I share a raunchy, vicious sense of humor and a history of intensive therapy and daily antidepressant cocktails, was my twin. Lindsay vacillated between being my older or my kid sister. In complicated, infuriating ways, I feel like Wendy was my daughter.

This is our story—mine, Katie's, Lindsay's, Mimi's, and Wendy's. Though not completely factual, it is the truth as we lived it.

I hope that you will learn something of the extreme effort of living fat and of dieting from our year of struggle. I hope that you will come away with more compassion or with self-forgiveness when nature wins out over intention. Most of all, I hope that more friendships come out of this book. When women come together in order to tell their stories and their truths, they become collectively strong in their individual weaknesses. That is the positive power of anger. It can open a me-too that we so rarely feel in the horrible loneliness of being fat or diffident dieting. We are none of us either the only one or alone.

ONE

April

Déjà Vu All Over Again

Here is the truth: one night I got into bed with Daisy, my yellow Labrador retriever, and Malachi, a goofy black Lab who was staying with us for a couple of cramped and restless nights. I had a pint of Ben & Jerry's chocolate chip cookie dough ice cream. I took a spoonful of the dough part for myself, then a spoon of the vanilla for Daisy and Mally. Mally made a mess of my quilt, but it was time to wash it anyway.

Two nights later I bought another pint of ice cream and shared it with my bedmates. After the second lick or so, Mally scraped the ice cream off the spoon with his front teeth.

No more melted ice cream dripping on the quilt.

I hadn't realized that Daisy ate ice cream by scraping it off the spoon, the way humans do, until our visiting galoot learned to do the same. I ran into Mally's owner a few days later and told him the story. A lightbulb floated over his head. "So *that's* why Mally went berserkers last night when I took a spoon out of the drawer!"

There were rules I lived by but couldn't say out loud. Like any functioning alcoholic or closet baser, I kept my addiction in check. One of my rules was not eating sugar during the day. It makes me drowsy and lazy, and because I walk dogs for a living, I need to be alert. Until I had a dog of my own and then three or four more young Labs to jerk me around, I didn't know the menace of the streets. There is a bloodthirsty Akita two blocks down, and there are chicken bones in gutters; joggers swing their arms crazily on the Promenade, and there are babies who don't understand dog kisses everywhere.

Another truth is that by not eating sugar during the day, there was a slight chance I wouldn't at night. In truth there is hope.

But after arguing with dogs, my hands rough from exposure to four months of winter, my back and hips aching, I spent my nights in the pacifying arms of Entenmann's, Ben & Jerry's, Cinnamon Life Cereal, European rice pudding, and the occasional order of Fascati's chicken Parmesan with garlic bread.

You'd think my awareness that eating makes me drunk and non-reactive, that my dog has learned to eat neatly from a spoon and fork, would be red flags for how indiscriminate my reasoning had become. It wasn't. Something as quiet and unfunny as a fact—a number—would have to knock me back to the truth of myself.

My résumé is full of facts that dance crazily across a contrary map of truth.

Take, for instance, the fulfillment of my lifelong desire to publish a book. I had no subject for a book until I lost 188 pounds, going from a size 32 to a size 6, after forty-two years of obesity. It was sold and published. Destroying the satisfaction I should have taken from years of my writing apprenticeship took cunning and craft.

But I did it. By the time I sat next to Bob Greene while Oprah grilled Winona Judd on the whys and hows of her rotundity, my upper arms and breasts felt like overstuffed sausage meat in my size 16 red velvet dress. I had terrible gas from the chocolate-covered almonds I'd eaten the night before and was full of resentment because sharing the green room with Bob Greene meant I didn't dare eat the pastries they provided for guests.

Needless to say, the camera did not turn to me for my thoughts on the matter.

My opinion would have made for terrible viewing. *You can lose weight, Winona*, I would have said, *but you'll gain it back.*

Still, I think that pontificating with Hoba Kotb on the *Weekend Today Show* about how much better my life was with 188 fewer pounds to heave around, then watching my Amazon rating go to twelve that afternoon while eating an entire key lime pie, is guerilla sabotage raised to a high art, don't you?

Some few weeks after the dogs' and my ice cream social, as March made its false promises, I house-sat two Italian greyhounds. As I waited for them to pick at their food, I wandered around the apartment looking at knickknacks and art choices and the absence of a bookcase. (I wasn't snooping, in case you wonder about dog walkers coming into your home. I have enough trouble with the privacies and troubles of my own life to creep into anyone else's.) There was a scale in the bathroom. While the dogs jetéed merrily around my feet, I decided to step onto the scale.

Foolish, foolish me.

The digital readout settled squarely at 250.

My one-hundred-pound gain cracked the air. Smoke curled from my toes where they framed the infamous number. The once-adoring greyhounds turned into creatures from Hieronymus Bosch swarmed up my legs like hungry accusing succubae. I'd ignored tsking mirrors and grouching body aches, but the scale spoke the fact.

One hundred pounds in three years. Before that, four years of dieting and maintaining, an adventure that commenced on March 9, 1998. That morning on the borrowed scale was March 11, 2006.

I had lost my body. In getting so big again, I had shrunk to planning the next binge. I stepped off the scale not as Frances Kuffel but as One Hundred Pounds in Three Years Kuffel.

I had only one option: I was going to have to rescramble the facts and lose this weight and, somehow, get my self back into living color.

I'd gotten thin through the confederacy of a twelve-step program I fondly call the "Stepfords." My original sponsors, Katie and Bridget, had moved away from New York, so when I saw the numbers on the scale, I called one of the last old-timers from the meetings, known by twelve-step members as the "Rooms," I habituated. Twenty years earlier, Patty had stopped fifteen years of vicious bulimia with the help of the Stepfords. She had the longest recovery of anyone left in the meetings I attended, although her largest size had been a mere eighteen.

Early in April, as I was beginning to interview women for this book, I dug up my Stepford phone list and called her. "You have to sponsor me."

"I don't really have time for more sponsees,"[5] she said. "I can take your food until you find a sponsor, though."[6]

"You don't understand. You are my sponsor now. You don't have a choice. You're the only person I know with the recovery and"—here my voice broke—"the kindness I need." I had gained weight by eating sugar and flour. I was, therefore, bad—immoral, in a state of mortal sin, as corrupt as the last four presidents combined—and I needed not only forgiveness but benevolence in order to mend my evil ways.

"Okay," she said, her voice softening, "can you call me at five fifteen tomorrow morning?"

In three minutes I was back in Program.[7]

---

5   A sponsee is twelve-step parlance for the person one sponsors through the recovery process of a food plan, weight loss, and working the twelve steps.

6   "Take your food" is specific to twelve-step programs for eating disorders. The sponsee "gives" his food (that is, reports it) to his sponsor each day. The sponsor, in return, "takes" it.

7   "Program" is more twelve-step jargon. It means the individual, no matter what addiction fellowship s/he is in, is following the suggested guidelines for staying away from behaviors

Twelve-step thinking tends to be black-and-white—you're clean[8] or you're not, and "clean" doesn't have much credibility until you have ninety days. The home meeting[9] I attended had changed. My posse had largely disbanded, and there wasn't much talk of weight loss. I'd been taught to keep my mouth shut for the first ninety days of abstinence, to listen rather than speak in meetings, where foods are never specified[10] and the emphasis is on "hope, strength, and experience." I had plenty of the latter but very little hope or strength.

A week into working with Patty, she told me to write a history of my relapse. I did so on my Amazon blog. It was a rambling thing but people responded, and those readers gave me the company and support that I'd been missing in my current life of windchills, dogs, sugar, and wobbling abstinence. Blogging also made me more real to myself.

Katie was deliberating on the practical matter of her suicide.

She had already chosen the date—May 29, six weeks away, both sensible and sensitive: her brothers and mother wouldn't have to remember separate dates for her fortieth birthday and her death.

That was easy, she thought as she slipped her fingers along the edges of a box of carrot cake. The top lifted at a forty-five-degree angle. She took a forkful of frosting from the edge of the cardboard platter and allowed her attention to wander to the subject of packaging. Was it possible that Entenmann's intended these fragile lids to

---

and substances. "Working a program" generally includes going to meetings, calling other members, doing twelve-step work, calling one's sponsor, and reading designated literature.

8   "Clean" means you are habitually eschewing certain foods.

9   A "home meeting" is a meeting one goes to weekly and considers most familiar.

10   Instead, one hears references to "that cold sweet stuff" or "the Italian take-out item."

dent like this so that consumers had no choice but to finish off the box in one go? "I wouldn't put it past them," she said to the living room wall, and kicked back in her La-Z-Boy. She stabbed into the cake and returned to the business of her death. Where she would do it was dictated by how, and how continued to dizzy her with possibilities.

She'd tried pills, and she certainly didn't want a repetition of the scenes with her family, the hospital, and shrinks that method had caused three years earlier. A gun would pretty much wipe out the good intentions of May 29, as would razor blades. In any case, neither had ever been serious options.

There was nothing cleaner than pulling a James Mason/Spalding Gray—should she take a drive over to Half Moon Bay? But such a dignified death was reserved for those who would *sink*. Katie would bob in with the tide and find it as hard to get off the shoreline as the proverbial beached whale. Hanging was also the province of the thin— she had visions of bringing down rafters and scaffolding. Throwing herself off some rooftop would flatten anyone or thing she fell on. She didn't have a garage, so carbon monoxide was a non-option.

The San Mateo Bridge was good—but would she be found?

That was a bad thought. Only crumbs and a scant rime of frosting were left of her cake. *Who will find me? Ingrid?* As if Ingrid didn't do enough listening as a psychotherapist, the poor woman had listened to her troubles for three years, listened to Katie at 140 pounds larding up to her most recent weigh-in, on a meat-packing scale, of 427. She couldn't do that to Ingrid, and because Katie had been fired from her Searles sales rep job the month before, it wasn't like anyone expected her to show up anywhere, except maybe her DBT classes.[11]

---

11 Dialectical Behavior Therapy was pioneered by Marsha Linehan at the University of Washington for the treatment of Borderline Personality Disorder. Linehan's thesis is that "an 'emotionally vulnerable' person . . . is someone whose autonomic nervous system reacts excessively to relatively low levels of stress and takes longer than normal to return to baseline once the stress is removed. It is proposed that this is the consequence of a

What would her teacher have to say of her student who gave in to her emotional mind over the supposed reasoning of her wise mind?

Probably that Katie had left an emotional corpse, but that the HMO had been wise for putting her in therapy and was therefore finished with a job well done.

That left dying at home in San Bruno and sending a letter to her mother in Sacramento, which made timing tricky. She'd have to do it before her mother could prevent it but not so early that her mother would find her all smelly and puddly.

Katie shuddered and opened a box of hot cross buns, appropriate for Lent and the fact that she was mourning for two, herself and Christianity.

More than anything, Katie wanted to have choices, and in a year in which her most favorite thing of all, theme cakes (there was nothing like a *bûche de Noël* or red velvet Valentine's Day cake with which to acknowledge a holiday going on outside her apartment), seemed to be on strike, carrot versus banana crunch cake was not a choice. There were no circles on the calendar Katie had not bothered to hang. A calendar meant dates to remember, a future to plan, choices to make between movies or job interviews. Carrot cake, German chocolate cake, coconut cake: they had chosen her, and one would follow upon the other as inevitably as breathing. Instinct would not stop her from eating or inhaling, and in pulling the curtains across the affable warmth of April, she had decided to decide what she could.

"She claimed her own life," Katie rehearsed for her hometown newspaper, grimly acknowledging the irony of her words. Death was an action, a choice, a future. She wanted those things more than she wanted a white sheet cake with green coconut frosting and hard sugar

---

biological diathesis." Barry Stearns and Michaela Swales, "An Overview of Dialectical Behavior Therapy in the Treatment of Borderline Personality Disorder," Psychiatry Online, http://www.priory.com/dbt.htm.

shamrocks. She wanted to own her death. She wanted to leave a corpse, and she wanted her family to know she'd done it while trying to protect their feelings. She wanted dignity, and the most dignified suicide she could think of was Ben Kingsley in his general's uniform, duct-taping a plastic bag around his neck with deft determination at the end of *House of Sand and Fog*.

If only she knew what kind of bag he'd used.

At that, she started to cry some more.

Mimi's knee was killing her. The coed on the Weight Watchers scale was asking a lot of questions about losing more quickly, and Mimi would gladly have smacked her if she could keep her place in the line. Surely the girl would know what was coming if she saw Mimi, stocky as a mushroom in black leggings and a red T-shirt, hobbling out of line and aiming straight for her. *Isn't being here torture enough?* she wanted to ask the twentysomething married-with-toddler suburbanite behind her. *I have a fifty-hour-a-week job, and you're raising a kid. Why does trying to lose weight have to be a second career?*

Mimi had skipped breakfast and water, and forgone her warm chenille tunic for this weigh-in on a Saturday morning when she could be preparing for the holidays coming up. That year, April was busier than Christmas, what with the full Pink Moon Esbat just before Easter, and Beltane Sabbat two weeks later. She could be sharing that divine coffee cake and chorizo omelet at the Union with Lilith, showing her one of the dogwood candles she had molded in the sand and pebbles of White Clay Creek. Lilith and her husband had invited Mimi to celebrate the dogwood by casting a circle of fertility, followed by a ritual hot tub, and Mimi needed fresh whole spices for cookies. With a yawn, she had thought about sleeping in. Her doctor had broached the possibility of supplementing her CPAP machine with sleep apnea medication, although she was kind enough to compliment Mimi on keeping her weight within twenty pounds for the last couple of years.

Not so her orthopedist. He had no compunction about informing her that she needed orthoscopy on her right knee this summer with the other to follow within two or three years if she didn't do something about her weight.

And so here she was, fifty-two years old, in line with a two-year-old whining behind her, and a college junior "wondering" if three pounds a week wasn't unreasonably slow, what with spring break coming up. Mimi knew the scale would do exactly what it wanted to, hovering a pound or three up or down from 255, but really, after delays at the Salt Lake airport en route from presenting at a PubMed class and the temptation of Cinnabon and Rocky Mountain Chocolate Factory, what did she expect?

At least I threw the last couple of chocolates out. If I just had more self-control, she thought for the thirty-sixth time that morning. *If I just gave up* one *thing. There must be life after chocolate . . .*

When her turn came, it was quick. "Two-five-four-point-two," Linda said, writing the numbers down in her log. "That's terrific, Mimi! A point-three-pound loss! Keep up the good work!"

Mimi smiled for Linda and thanked her. That could add up to a whopping fifteen-point-something loss in a year, by golly. *I could be at goal weight when I'm five-seven-point-something years old!*

It was eleven o'clock on a cloudy and cold but dry Saturday in April when the meeting was over and they'd gotten their new recipes and reminders about drinking water. Mimi decided to turn her hunger and sarcasm into optimism and head for Whole Foods with Linda's three-point turtle "cheesecake" recipe in hand.

We who eat compulsively, eat instead of speaking. We are the stars in a play for one actor, and both the stage and the dialogue are our bodies for the rare, critical audience. Like great drama, weight is showing, not telling, a psychic and biological story.

Losing weight is the opposite of the dumb show of gain. The

audience is bigger, more varied, and more vocal. Confessions are made ("I have issues with food, too," my internist, who had hectored me about my obesity, admitted when I lost weight. Could she have told me that a hundred pounds of fat, despair, and confusion earlier???) and ambitions are formed.

The impulse to lose doesn't always involve three-digit numbers, fantasies, or the demands of doctors. It is not always epic. Sometimes weight loss is the drama of facing what is under our beds or behind the curtains, ferreting out the icky sources of unhappiness we furthered by our eating. We are in search of the courage to no longer ignore our dreams and to demand that we be taken seriously as we fashion a fitter, more disciplined body. These are fundamental principles in an authentic life.

Lindsay slapped the snooze bar one more time and twisted the pillow under her ear. Why get up when she could hear the shower running? One of the things Jalen couldn't stand was her peeing when he was using the bathroom.

Jalen woke her before she got her seven minutes' grace from *Morning Edition*. He sat down heavily on her side of the bed and said, "Look at my blister."

Lindsay mumbled concerned noises and burrowed deeper into the comforter.

"It's worse today."

"Mmm."

"I could barely keep running after seven miles."

"Awww."

"It really hurts, Linds. What am I gonna do? We're running Fuller Park to Tannery tonight."

Lindsay summoned up a complete sentence at last. "Skip it, Easton."

"Hon," he said in that reasoning-but-really-whining voice that felt like a forklift. "I can't skip it. I got the okay from the parks department for the run." Jalen was good at coming up with plans for his running club. He was also good at coming up with basketball and tennis courts, baseball diamonds and swimming lanes. Lindsay was good at coming up with another seven minutes of sleep.

"Linds, wake up. I'm gonna lance it, and then I want you to bandage it."

Lindsay sighed and threw off the covers. He wouldn't leave her alone, so she might as well get up.

Jalen saw her emerging from the quilt and stood up.

"Tell me honestly, hon. Do I look fat?"

She groaned. He asked the question every morning and every night, and she groaned each time.

"You weigh less than I do, Jay. Stop it."

The thing about weighing thirty—*thirty!*—pounds more than your husband is that you never get to ask that specific question. You're stuck with variations on "Does this make me look fat[ter]?" or "Do you love my body?"

She could hear a jazz combo between segments of the radio program as she went through her morning routine. The music was redolent of smoky little nightclubs and shiny red nail polish, and she clenched her fists thinking of her ragged cuticles. She pulled off her flannel nightgown and scowled at how her tummy flamed over her hips, then stepped on the scale, telling herself that if the readout wasn't less than the 172 that she'd held on to through the last two weeks of no wine, no popcorn at night, no lattes, and regular workouts, she'd bump her three-mile run up to five for the next couple of days. She took a deep breath as she hesitated. Jalen would notice if she increased her running. He would bite his tongue not to give advice, making the air heavy. There would certainly be an invitation to go along with his club, which meant a choice between hurting his feelings or coming home crazed from watching him run in tandem with Patra Fletch, his partner in Home Fit, their personal trainer company—if two people could be called a company.

It was one thing to do a leisurely jog around Tinker's Creek on a cool sunny April Sunday, admiring Jalen's gorgeousness and the sprinkles of buttercups. It was another thing to join his crew as one of the slower of the dozen.

Patra Fletch was not slower. She was a prodigy of self-sculpture. *With a name like that, just wouldn't she be?* Lindsay asked the mirror. Her red delicious apple cheeks and her ponytail bobbed back at her in agreement. Lindsay had a moment of admiring her ponytail, enough to step on the scale. The numbers flashed and settled on 171.4. Her first fear about Jalen was over for the day.

Dieting is scientific and mechanical: fewer calories expended than consumed day after day after goddammed day.

The semantics of dieting, on the other hand, are about as exacting as playing an étude wearing oven mitts. This concerns me because failure is built into the semantics.

This linguistic sloppiness starts in the secret of our heart. "I have to do something about my weight," Mimi was telling herself as she floundered with Weight Watchers. The statement is a stalling tactic, hinged on the words "do something." Mimi is not stupid. She has a master's degree in medical library science and holds a prestigious job. If "do something" meant working to get the flab off her body, she'd be speaking in specifics: "I have to go back to the Weight Watchers Core Plan" or "I have to stop eating gelato." "Do something" can mean anything. I could, for instance, paint my weight in silver and gold glitter or sing about it. The phrase has nothing to do with intention, but as long as we say we have to do something about it, we're—maybe— fooling ourselves and others that we're on the brink of, um, a diet.

Then, of course, there are the questions.

"How did you lose the weight?"

The weight? The use of the definite article instead of a pronoun separates fat from the person in question, either as a form of sensitivity or a refusal to understand that the fat body was and continues to be as much a part of the person as her thinner body.

The also turns weight into community property, the way a wife might ask her husband, "How did you lose the keys?" as they stand in the rain outside their locked car. "Lose" is problematic, too. To lose something is to hope to find it.

Is there one big stockpile of fat that we all draw on? Is there a Fat Lost and Found at which we have to describe our weight ("It's thigh fat, about thirty inches, with dimples?") in order to reclaim it?

If I lose property that is exclusively mine, the noun is preceded by a personal pronoun: "How did you lose your book report, Frances?"

There is nothing more personally and exclusively mine than the weight I bear. It is a more conscious and public part of me than my joy or sexuality or great hair. My weight or my size crosses my mind every time I make a meal, make a date, bend over to tie my shoes, go outside, put on clothes, and countless other motions and imaginings.

The word *weight* in that question is just as peculiar. The most successful anorectic has weight, a glimmer of a fetus has weight. Without a qualification (even a generic one such as "so much weight") and taken literally, talking about losing weight reduces the successful dieter to nothing at all. Further, *weight* says nothing of what, really, weight *is*. Weight is muscle and bones and blood and organs and fat. We don't burn weight, we burn fat, from which getting thinner is a by-product. Is fat so alien, so unmentionable, that it's safer to talk about it in terms of sterility and separateness, an item made of not-us? Still, the question of how, unreflective as it is, persists. As it happens, the Angry Fat Girls put their money where their mouths are in two organizations. Katie and I have continued our alliance with twelve-step programs for eating disorders, and Wendy, Mimi, and Lindsay attend Weight Watchers. Our organizations do not dictate the how of dieting, there aren't necessarily set perimeters. Our food varies from day to day, and each camp has its own vocabulary for operating within it.

The lingo that twelve-step programs for eating disorders employ is as wide of the mark as any other. "I've given away fifty pounds," you might hear a particularly enthusiastic member say. "To whom," I want to snap, "a thirteen-year-old anorectic?" The newly thin would answer that she gave her pounds to God or HP, "Higher Power," just as she turns over all of her life to Him or Her or It. I can't bear people talking about HP. I inevitably wonder how Hewlett-Packard has provided a miracle.

"I've released fifty pounds," another twelve-stepper might say. This is somewhat more realistic except that it's backwards, isn't it? Wouldn't fifty fewer pounds release the body?

Ought we say, "I have been *relieved* of fifty pounds"?

Or our inquisitors could frame the question of how someone loses weight the way they might ask how someone eased another physical ailment: "How did you get rid of your migraines?" or "How did you cure your flu?"

At least these questions aren't hinting that we will re-find our weight or that it, like Lassie, will re-find us, which is found in that announcement that, yes, we'll have dessert, but "I just hope it doesn't show up on the scale tomorrow," as though the needle will bounce around until it settles on cheesecake.

Members of twelve-step programs for eating disorders speak of their food as being "clean" and "tight" in addition to the broad generalization of "abstinent," which means whatever the going definition of refraining from compulsive eating is.[12]

Members "work a strong Program" and participation is complicated. As a Stepford Wife, I can attest that Program requires a lot of time and something between obedience and surrender, as stated in the

---

12 Some twelve-step programs ban particular foods and chemicals, and have exact measurements and rules around sanctioned food. Other programs do not mandate a particular plan of eating.

source for all of the 601 twelve-step programs, *Alcoholics Anonymous.*[13] "Those who do not recover are people who *cannot* or *will not completely* give themselves to this *simple* program ... "[14] There are meetings to attend, calls to make, histories to be written, amends to make to people we have harmed, books beyond the Big Book to be read.

Weight Watchers, which itself is a brand name open to interpretation (someone who is "watching his weight" is usually trying either to maintain his weight or lose a few, rather than a lot of, pounds. Or does the weight watcher watch his weight the way birders observe the Bicknell's thrush?), offers two diet plans, the Flex and the Core plans. The names probably say it all, but Flex allows the greatest variety of foods, each of which is assigned a certain number of points. The Core Plan, which doesn't use points, relies on the Core List of foods, which are basically fresh, unprocessed foods and do not include any breads. Denise, a responder to my blog who uses the Flex Plan, instructed someone who asked about Weight Watchers, "You are supposed to eat as much of the Core foods as it takes to feel 'satisfied,' which is the scary part of that option. Who is ever satisfied when it comes to food? If I knew that feeling, would I have a weight problem to begin with ... ?"

No counting? How can you lose weight without counting? If you don't count calories (or points), you're going to have to count something else. Ounces. Cups. Units.

Weight Watchers is the most lucrative company in the fifth-largest industry in our economy, generating $50 billion a year. In 2003, Weight Watchers' revenue was approximately $943 million, while Jenny Craig saw $280 million and LA Weight Loss achieved

---

13   Most often referred to as the Big Book.

14   Alcoholics Anonymous, 3rd ed. (Alcoholics Anonymous World Services: N.p., 1986), 58. The italics reflect how the passage is read out loud.

$250 million in gross income.[15] Their revenues are higher yet when special supplements and branded foods are added.

Diet programs are not cheap. According to *Forbes*, the first week in Weight Watchers, in which one pays initiation fees and shops for new foods in order to follow the Flex Plan, costs $385. If the average American household spends $5,781 a year on food, this breaks down to about $27.79 a week per person, exclusive of fast food.[16] Diets culled from books rather than organizations are equally expensive. Following *21 Pounds in 21 Days: The Martha's Vineyard Diet Detox* calls for a $200 kit of supplements, a juicer, weekly visits to a colon therapist, and organic foods.

Successful dieting relies on devout dieters, and the various programs have their own scriptures, saints, forms of worship, and accountability to some kind of authority, whether it's a food journal, a weekly weigh-in, or Weight Watchers' online POINTS Tracker with its twenty-seven thousand foods. Lindsay designed her own computer program, using the Weight Watchers Flex Plan points and the calorie deductions of her exercise regime, and one of our readers' husband designed a computer spreadsheet program based on protein/carbohydrates/fats.

Programs, regimes, spreadsheets?

Then again, there's always the "Unrequited Love Weight Loss Method."

I'm hungry, Wendy thought as she practiced pull-ups in the shallow end of the pool.

With that, she breathed in a large stream of water, proving that

---

15   Ellen Goodstein, "10 Secrets of the Weight-Loss Industry," Bankrate.com, February 2, 2005 (accessed).

16   Rebecca Ruiz, "How Expensive Is Your Diet?" ABC News, January 2, 2008, http://abcnews.go.com/Business/PersonalFinance/story?id=4086537&page=1.

humans can scream under water. Marilyn, her instructor, waded over to help steady her while she sputtered and coughed.

"What happened?" Marilyn asked. "What made you panic?"

Wendy was still clearing water from her nose, making her accent more Southern and her voice as atonal as if she had a cold. "I lost my concentration." Her heart broke open for the eighty-second time that day. Wendy had to remind herself that this wasn't Marilyn's problem.

"Why don't you try the crawl over to the fourth lane and then pull up from it," Marilyn suggested. "If you have more to concentrate on, you won't lose your feet."

She meant well, Marilyn did. This was Wendy's third terrified swimmer's class with Marilyn, and she didn't almost drown very often anymore. She trusted Marilyn with her life the first time she put her face in the water and ended up sitting on the edge of the pool crying and shaking.

Wendy was rattled to her core. Her mind was on Five Continents and their warm, fresh tortilla chips. At the same time, she could feel her nose and chin tingling, the first sign she was fighting the water and a blasting body memory of that first class and Cal's sucker punch to her heart seventeen days ago.

Wendy left her husband, Leo, in November of 2004, after one last argument concerning his love for her but complete lack of sexual desire for anyone. Out of habit, they went to her parents' house for Thanksgiving, but by mid-December, Wendy was actively looking for a New Year's Eve date. The habits of her twenty-year marriage quickly dribbled out.

She spent New Year's Eve with her friend from the enrollment office, Susan, but she vowed the next year would be different.

It was and it wasn't. Wendy is the supreme postponer: she and Leo were no closer to divorce than they'd been fifteen months earlier. She'd started dating Cal, but he had kids and their 2006 New Year's Eve was phone sex.

Cal was boyfriend heaven. They were good together, she protested to herself for the millionth time. Okay, as Madeline pointed out, he had his kids on weekends and an ex-wife he continued to perform honey-do's for. He was a mechanic; he wasn't going to get any richer, and he wasn't anywhere near rich now. He hadn't gone to college, didn't read, liked eighties pop music. But Cal was a big man, over six feet tall, muscles running a little to fat, swarthy and black-haired with a big handlebar mustache. For the first time she didn't feel like she dwarfed a guy. He was handy when stuff like her three-year-old Honda Civic and her Mac notebook went bonkers. All of that amounted to a feeling of being protected and taken care of, a feeling she hadn't had since before the rebellions of puberty when her daddy did everything he could to keep his little girl from getting hurt.

She was left with questions she couldn't avoid. How many women had he cheated with? It took her three months of believing his excuses and lies before she actually tracked him down at *her* house. Such a fucking idiot! He sent Carol downstairs with the excuse that she had children and wouldn't tolerate a scene, then he packed Wendy off to visit her childhood friend Madeline in Athens, Georgia. He promised that he'd break up with the bitch while she was gone. "We'll get past this, babe. Trust me. You know me. You know how much I want you."

On Sunday morning, as Madeline was brewing coffee and making cinnamon toast, Wendy checked her email and found what she was sure would be Cal's description of the explosion with Carol.

> You know I can't stand to see you cry. But, I've damaged us too much. I don't think you'd ever trust me again & I don't know how I could make up what I done to you. It's not that I love Carol, but she lets me be me and right now I need a positive person in my life. She has kids. She understands what it's like for me, being a single dad & all. You'll meet some smart guy real soon who has his act together and who has more in common with you than I. Please don't take this personally. It's just bad timing.

She'd emailed him back immediately, which she now regretted. If she'd waited, she could have kept him on pins and needles and then been *really* cutting, she thought as she plodded toward the locker room: *Does she understand that your kids think she's dumb as a box of rocks? Does she get that you cheat left and right? Does either of you know* any *rules of grammar?*

Wendy was amazed that one body could hold so many tears. Madeline had kept her well supplied with reefer, vodka, busyness, and insults, nicknaming Cal "Idiot Man" and Carol "She-Male," but the return to Williamsburg sent Wendy crashing. One thing about having a nervous breakdown out of town with your best friend, she realized, is that you can say I'll have cheese dip with that.

Wearing her bra and underwear, Wendy padded over to the locker room scale, slid the top weight to 273. The end remained in place until she tapped it to 272.

Another pound lost. Cal was good for something after all. Her best friend in Williamsburg, Susan, had been begging her to go to Weight Watchers with her. Maybe *they* could tell her what to eat when she was too sad to figure it out for herself.

Wendy was not alone in wondering what she could eat that would end her obesity. In 2006, the *Washington Post* reported that about 62 percent of American women were overweight or obese,[17] while 80 percent of American women think they are overweight.[18]

In regaining weight, we (and 95 percent of us who lose weight will regain it, and more, within five years) betray the labor, struggle,

---

17 Rob Stein, "Obesity Among U.S. Women Leveling Off, Study Shows," April 5, 2006.

18 Theresa Makin, "Truth in Advertising," *The Harvard Salient*, May 6, 1999.

financial investment, and newfound hopes about ourselves.[19] We unearthed time to go to meetings, buy and chop eggplants, sweat on treadmills, read books and labels and recipes instead of tearing open bags and boxes. We who blamed our obesity on laziness and lack of willpower obeyed programs and nutritionists and sponsors and personal trainers as though we were assembling the trickiest of Ikea bookcases.

That, in fact, is precisely what we were doing, making new pieces of furniture by taming our bodies. In the years it took to lose 275 or 190 or 100 pounds, we accumulated new hardware; our toolboxes included determination, commitment, hope, goals, shy pride, and self-possession as we said "no" to wedding cake and "help me" to experts and "does this fit?" to clerks in misses' departments. We became bodies and characters we didn't know but had spent our lives thinking about other women. *She's beautiful. She's so disciplined. I wish I could get away with wearing that. How does she do it?*

And then, our self-invented strengths and bodies became bookcases that wobbled more every day. We were living fraudulently in our different bodies and our different ways of eating until the bookcase splintered apart.

That April, the cruelest month, when memory mixes with desire, we realized the facts of our thinness could not support the weighty truth of us.

---

19   Sharon Dalton, *Overweight and Weight Management* (Boston: Jones and Bartlett Publishers, 1997), 396.

TWO

May

The Unbearable Being of Lightness

It was a hundred degrees at two p.m. in Arizona, where I was visiting my parents that May. My Amazon blog was thriving as I wrote a brief entry from my parents' bedroom computer. Over the next three days, there were nineteen responses or, more aptly, conversations. Spring cleaning and gardening, Pilates and exercise were on everyone's mind as they enjoyed the seventy-degree weather beyond the blinding desert, and they were trading tips on breathing and yoga.

Lindsay wrote about trying not to panic over defending her dissertation proposal and finding relief, as she always did, in doing something physical. "I got rid of this big ugly bush this weekend. It was something I'd hacked at here and there for the last five years. I cut it down, and it looks so much better. I've been telling the story as the Parable of the Ugly Bush, as in, it was not in that bush's nature to be anything but ugly. It wasn't the bush's fault, it wasn't my fault. It just looked ugly and scratched the hell out of me every time I had to deal with it." She didn't say what the parable meant, but it could easily have applied to our struggles with weight.

Mimi was dealing with doctors regarding her arthritic knees, sleep apnea, and a diabetes scare. "I can be overweight and healthy, or I can be overweight and unhealthy. I want to be healthy regardless of what my weight is and that means sucking it up and having the tests and hearing harsh truths," she wrote. The blog gave her a safe place to talk about the doctors and her history of obesity, her family's concern, and the physical pain she was in—and to recognize that she was in emotional pain over these things. "Today, right now, I can deal with it, but some days I just can't and it makes me cry and retreat into myself. I think I'll take the rest of the day off, go outside, and walk barefoot in the grass and celebrate the fact the spring is finally apparently here. It's taken forever."

Wendy wrote that she was getting out of the top women's sizes, but her elation was mixed with ennui. "I am sitting here [at work] tired, sad, and I want to go home and rest and reread the WW booklets and come up with a plan."

At the time, Lindsay, Mimi, and Wendy were just three responders among others. I certainly didn't think any of them would become my closest friends.

Katie didn't contribute to the blog that day but I later found out that in May she had gone back to OA, Overeaters Anonymous, and found a sponsor. She was no longer suicidal and had realized she didn't want to die so much as she wanted to get her family's attention and compassion.

The readers of my Amazon blog needed the space I created, but they didn't need me, which was fine. I was absorbed in my own life, walking dogs and doing research for this book, my ongoing confusion about what Scott—known as the Boy from Connecticut in *Passing for Thin*—and I were doing on the phone for hours every day at the same time that I was casually seeing and sleeping with another man. I was glad to see so much activity, but I have to admit I didn't feel the same warmth for these women as they did for each other.

Largely blind to what was happening, I merely smiled at Wendy playing the hostess. "Welcome," she wrote to a newcomer who was mystified by the whole Amazon-blog thing. "We talk a lot here." Nor did I notice when Mimi wrote to Wendy, "I'm sorry you're sad. But rereading the WW booklets is a good thing. We can come up with a plan together, how's that? And yes, I have IM and I'd *love* to visit with you that way! I'll send you my name."

In the same stream of responses to the short entry I wrote on May 4, Wendy wrote to another responder, "It's true that we all seem to have a lot in common. Let me figure out a way to link a survey and we can have fun with statistics. (Or is that an oxymoron?)"

The Angry Fat Girls were born while I was in Sun City, Arizona, biting my nails in boredom and fear of my parents' advancing age.

A long conversation broke out about whether there is a caste system for the obese. Lia's position was beautifully articulated: "I think it's more of a class system. Movement within a caste system is a lot harder than movement within a class system, and that's one of the scariest things about being overweight—it's a lot easier to move up (down) than it is to maintain your status."

I heaved a sigh when I read that, thinking back three years to another return from Arizona to New York and the chain of events that led to the unraveling of my maintenance and my self.

I hadn't yet sat down at my desk when the telephone rang.

"How are you, Frances?" my boss, Alix, asked in a voice more cheerful than I'd heard in months. "How was the conference? How were your parents?"

It was a Wednesday, my first day back from a writers' conference and short visit with my parents in Arizona. "The conference was good," I said, "and my parents are pretty well, considering."

"Why don't you make yourself a cup of tea and come in and join me?"

Humph, I thought. *She's barely spoken to me since the blowup and now she wants to have morning tea together?* Ignoring a pile of phone messages, I grabbed a legal pad to take dictation or make a list of things she wanted "us" to do.

"Shut the door," she said. I sat down in the chair angled away from the view of Central Park twenty-nine floors below. It was distracting, and I found it hard enough to make sense of what Alix said.

I uncapped my pen as she flipped open her own legal pad. "I am sorry to say that your services will no longer be required at this agency. There is no good purpose in prolonging our association." She popped a Nicorette between a molar and her cheek, looking rather like a pounce-ready dilophosaurus, and watched for my reaction. When I gave none, she pressed, as she always did, her questions a long finger-nail scratching to catch me off guard or overreactive. "What do you have to say?"

I gawped as I scrambled for what I was feeling, then said, with eerie, momentary calm, "Relieved that I will never have to sit across from this desk again."

If you read this scene carefully, you can see that articulating emotions comes slowly to me. I may experience an ache in my throat or gut, and I cry easily, but I can't always tell you whether it's anger or grief, nervousness or defensiveness. It's not unusual for me to need a couple of weeks to have names for my responses.

My reticence is dormancy, however, not stupidity. Like Yellow-stone's Mastiff Geyser, I erupt infrequently, briefly, but at 202 degrees and thirty feet in the air.

A few weeks before I was fired, I found a note attached to one of my clients' book contracts. "Please write a letter and send," it said in a coworker's handwriting.

Customarily, Alix signed cover letters for contracts, including those of my clients, but in the beginning of our two years together, I signed those letters. I couldn't remember when she took over the contract cover letters, and she had never stated this as a policy change as she did, for instance, forbidding flip-flops in the office. The agency was the Queen of Hearts's croquet ground. Any Alice who wandered in would think it bizarre that we were painting rosebushes red, but we never knew whose head would roll next.

I looked at Abigail nervously. "Did Alix ask me to write a letter for her to sign, or does she want me to sign and send it?"

"She said for you to do the letter and send," Abigail answered.

"Are you sure?"

"That's what she said. I wrote it down verbatim."

So I did and included a CC of the letter in the folder I gave her at the end of the day so she could keep apprised of the various projects I'd tended.

The next morning I found the copy of the letter on my desk with an angry scrawl.

We will discuss.

"We will discuss" were never good words from Alix.

The Mastiff Geyser percolated rapidly into action. When Alix arrived, an hour later, I was loaded for bear.

"Alix," I said, meeting her in the hall and flapping the letter, "the note attached to the contract told me to write the cover letter and send the contract. I double-checked this with Abigail."

"I don't want to discuss it now, Frances."

"But I do. I'm *sick* of never knowing what is policy and what isn't, of not knowing what I can and can't do. This is just one more damned thing I'm in trouble for because your directions weren't clear to either Abigail or me."

"Not now, Frances."

"Then when?"

"I'll call you."

I turned back to my office, shutting the door to sit, doubled over, breathing hard, trying not to cry. It was a cloudy day. Not much light filled my north-facing office. I rarely turned on the overhead light, preferring the imagined anonymity of sitting in the small pool of my desk lamp. The gray swath of sky behind me, which matched Alix's color scheme throughout the office, filled my veins. I felt trapped.

An hour later, the conversation quickly dwindled to the number of angels dancing on the nib of her Renzetti fountain pen.

"This has been always been procedure," she insisted.

"Would you like me to bring copies of cover letters I've sent my clients in the past?"

She laughed, sarcastically. "You've never signed a cover letter."

"*Bull*shit, Alix! You *raved* about the letter I sent with Hyacinth's contract."

She chewed the inside of her lip, considering this. That had been my biggest sale. "We made a mistake. I want it known as company policy that *I* sign all contract letters. Add it to the office manual and don't let this happen again."

"I *didn't* let it happen again. Abigail took your instructions down word-for-word. We're always taking letters and notes verbatim only to be told we did a terrible job later. Do you have any fucking idea what it's like to try to work when everything you do is either wrong or subject to change?"

"Add it to the manual, Frances. I don't want to discuss this any further."

That was the second time in my two years with Alix that I'd exploded. The first time, I ran out of the office hyperventilating in an octave I didn't know I could reach.

Having eaten instead of living with my feelings for most of my life, it's an onerous task to sort out my reactions. I'm pretty clear about things like heartbreak and love, but strong outward emotions—such as fury and desire—and the middle ground of disappointment, being teased, and preserving boundaries—is shrouded in a fog of inexperience. Despite being Alix's executive vice president, I couldn't be evenhanded about that contract because I hadn't questioned the shift in procedures when it first occurred. I couldn't establish a working rapport because of the precedents of subservience I set up when I *asked* to go to the dentist or on vacation or to a funeral instead of *telling* her I was going. I especially had not told her that it was inappropriate to touch me. Put a couple of glasses of wine in Alix, and she was twisting my nose, stamping on my feet, insisting I hold her around the waist and hip bump in time to music. She did these things in front of our staff, colleagues, and clients. The hip-bumping incident got us thrown out of an important party.

"If we worked for Simon & Schuster," I used to joke, "she'd be *so* fired."

Within forty-eight hours of one of these scenes, I would be summoned to a meeting and told I was on the verge of being fired. It was classic hangover regrets and I knew it and I was too scared to confront any one part of it. I needed the job and Alix owned the company. What could I do?

Writing about this episode in my life is exquisitely painful because, years later, every time I binge, I dream of Alix or my former boss, Barbara. Before moving to Alix's agency, I had worked within the irksomeness of being an outsider in Barbara's family business, but it was nothing compared to the lack of oxygen in my shiny office twenty-some floors above Central Park. Barbara had encouraged the cultivation of promising authors, and she felt a lifetime commitment to them. Alix was interested in nursing advances but not talent, and she could be ruthless in terminating writers. I hadn't been happy in either agency, but it couldn't be dumb coincidence: surely, I was to blame?

I was to blame. I wasn't a very good agent. Agents have to be ambitious. I wasn't. The big advances that make agents successful don't always make the writer successful, or not in the long run. I was content with smaller advances that the author had a reasonable chance of earning back, which would make a second book sale much more likely.

(In fact, I instructed my own agent to be cautious in her ambitions for the sale of *Passing for Thin* for exactly this reason.) Such thinking was counterintuitive to these successful entrepreneurs who supported families on 15 percent rather than the salary I received. And I was burning out on the reading and demanding clients and disappointments that are inherent in the job.

It didn't matter that I'd been fired with three months' severance, with my own book to finish and publicize. I'd wanted to be a writer as much as I'd wanted to be thin, but everything "good" (interesting, intelligent, sociable, diligent, passionate, sensitive, funny—*hireable*) about me had been a false front waiting to topple. It had finally happened. My fifteen-year career was a fake.

My body, at 150 pounds, felt equally fake—borrowed or stolen, unfamiliar and unexplored. Did both counterfeits have to shatter simultaneously?

In the months after being fired, I flopped around trying to invent a new me, doing anything not to think about how I should have hissed, mid-nose-twisting, *Don't you* ever *do that again,* to Alix, and trying anything that might keep me from eating.

I drifted, the invisible witness of the changeover in my wealthy Brooklyn neighborhood, picking up coffee as the Yups went to work, going to the store as the nannies and housekeepers and landscapers arrived, reading at Starbucks as the courthouse bureaucrats thronged Montague Street for lunch, heading to a twelve-step meeting as young bankers morphed into parents and the nannies crowded into the Mac store.

What to do, who to be? In those long days around the summer solstice, I was bereft of what slender sense of identity I'd had, stricken by the confirmation that I was, first, last, always fireable.

"Hi, Frances, how are you?"

"Fireable, thank you, and you?"

"What color are your eyes?"

"Fireable."

I was a marked woman. I might as well have been wearing a T-shirt with a scarlet *F* across my chest.

Alas, I am not as noble as Hester Prynne.

"The idea of you interviewing me is very sexy."

I found his voice very sexy.

"Would you boss me around?"

"You start to sit down across from my desk. I tell you to remain standing."

"Mmm," he said, his voice smooth as ghee. "What are you wearing?"

"A suit. A long skirt with a slit to the back of my knees."

"You have very sexy knees."

"This is *my* interview. We're here to find out if *you* have sexy knees."

"Tell me what to do."

I give great phone, my voice deep and a little rasty, as we say back in my native Montana, from smoking. It charmed authors and editors. Now I used it to charm boys with fantasies of older women knocking their thirtysomething egos around. If they wanted me, these younger men, then maybe fireable would recede. Maybe I'd have reason not to punish myself with food.

Slut Boys disappear quickly, back to being real—students or boyfriends or professors or potters. It was a double abandonment, of me and of my trial-sized identity as slut.

I looped-de-looped with food. "Why shouldn't I have a blackberry pie?" I asked a friend one morning. "How often is blackberry pie available? I'll get it out of my system, and it'll be over."

And so a blackberry pie and a pint of Häagen-Dazs would disappear in one sitting, and I'd take three Sominex to sleep through meals, fasting twenty-four hours, waking to something else I needed to eat or seduce out of my system.

One May weekend, when the wisteria was thick and the air sweet with roses, I slept with a man I wasn't sure I liked. In the middle of fucking me, he asked, breathlessly, "Will you agent my next book?"

"Will you blurb mine?" I asked back. He smiled sweetly, but his eyes said no and silence hung between us, hot and overused as the air in my apartment. Over lunch I learned he was married, a boundary I'd sworn not to cross. The day went from bad to worse, ending with him staying overnight when he hadn't intended to.

He fell heavily asleep as I lay awake, hating the invasion of my small space, debating who I disliked more, him or me. I listened to him snore, trapped under his arm and unable to turn over in bed. Finally, I got up, dressed, and went to an all-night deli on Clark Street. I bought a pint of Ben & Jerry's Limited Edition Oatmeal Cookie Dough Ice Cream—hey, limited edition, right? It would soon be unavailable, and anyway, I'd be abstinent in a day or two.

I sat down on a stoop to eat it, but it was frozen too hard for the flimsy spoon the clerk had thoughtfully provided. I went home, slid a real spoon from the kitchen cupboard, shut myself in the bathroom, and sat down on the laundry bag in the dark. It was as close to an orgasm as I was going to get that day.

My Amazon blog turned this sour day into a thing too many of us had shared not to laugh at in retrospect. "Eating while hiding in the bathroom sucks. Eating while hiding in your OWN bathroom sucks even more," I wrote and M. added, "I've been there, hiding in the bathroom, and yes, it's creepy. It goes to show to what lengths this addiction will take us."

I was hanging on to one new dream. My parents had returned to Montana after their winter in Arizona and my mother was reading the classified ads for litters of Labrador retrievers that would be available when I went home that August. She raised Labs when I was little and would pick out a winner for me, help me housebreak it, and get me started on the great adventure of finally having a dog.

Unfortunately, Montana is the birthplace of my compulsive eating and the last place on earth I could regain my abstinence. The yellow peasant loaf–sized baby we picked out turned out to be a stubborn, human-flesh-eating brat. I couldn't leave Daisy with my elderly parents, and I couldn't take her to the beach before she even knew her own name, let alone liked me enough to learn to come when called. Suddenly I was imprisoned with this adorable monster that hated being held (*crash!* there went one dream) and had actual tantrums.

Two scenes stand out in my mind from that summer. One is of scooping Daisy up in my arms and running to the bathroom with the liquid bowels of half a box of laxatives, holding the puppy as I shit so that she wouldn't take her own dump on the carpet.

The other is of standing at the kitchen sink, looking into the old apple tree heavy with fruit and bowed to the deck, while shoving a package of molasses cookies, one whole cookie after another, down my throat. *I am sorry to say*—gulp—*your services will no longer*—gulp—*be needed.* Those cookies set a precedent. That voice, the way Alix chewed the inside of her lip as she waited for me to justify this or that thing I hadn't known she wanted, her giggle when she wanted to impress a client or important editor—scenes real or pulled from possibility continue to haunt my dreams when my food is out of control.

Six weeks later, I returned to Brooklyn with Daisy and forty pounds I didn't have when I boarded the plane in Newark. What being fired hadn't taken from me, food had reclaimed. Thoroughly in its thrall, I have been a whore for it, a thief, a liar, a magician, a juggler, a soldier, and a spy. Each of these roles had a different relationship with food, the world of things, and the world of people. If this story seems like so much navel-gazing, consider the analysis I'm forced to go through in sorting it out. Jesus, with which self do I start?

This compulsion has been my best friend, whipping post, lover, and god since the age of three or four. It has ruined my ability to be automatically generous with others. My sense of my own worth, my health, my confidence, my discipline (clouded as it was by the fixation on and/or the sleepiness of food), my market value have been mown down by it even as food promised one more night of comfort against all those shortcomings. I was no longer an agent, no longer thin, no longer attractive as a slut, my German Slut Boy informed me. I was the owner of an energetic dog, in possession of a diagnosis of clinical depression and anxiety attacks when I had to leave the Bat Cave (what I called my small, dark apartment), and, if not a writer, an author.

There were grand moments and terrible ones in the next three years, variations on these themes of being fireable, inept, a liar when speaking about weight loss. My body bobbed up and down between 190 and 220 pounds, and my moods bobbed in tandem despite big doses of Zoloft, Wellbutrin, and when I developed problems breathing when I had to leave my house, Klonopin.

It was noon on a Saturday in January 2006, in a colorless church basement. It was a popular meeting, so the circle of Stepfords was large and not everyone would get his or her three minutes to talk about eating and life. For now, it was Rachel's turn.

"I haven't lost any weight in a long time," she said. I slid down in my chair, pulling my down coat closer. The big room was cold but the Michelin design of my outfit might confound anyone comparing me to her. We were about the same size.

"I don't think this program is doing me any good anymore," she went on. I looked at her from the corners of my eyes. "Whether I come or not, I follow my nutritionist's plan. I stay the same size; nothing is happening to my weight. In the meanwhile, I'm initiating a lawsuit against a boss and I need other fellowships to get through it."

When she smiled, Rachel was pretty, with unsuspected dimples and a bit of glee in her eyes. That Saturday she looked pale and drawn. Her skin showed old acne pits, and the scar of her harelip was a vivid childhood remnant of family troubles running deep and frightening through her nights.

"I'm sorry to hear you're having legal troubles," I said walking over to her after the Serenity Prayer. "Aren't you working on your own now?"

"Yeah," she said, "this is my ex-boss. I took a lot of verbal abuse from him."

I sat down at that.

"Really? Are you suing him or the company?"

"He is the company."

"Can you tell me a little about suing a boss? My ex-boss used to hit me in public, and it got to the point that I was scared to do anything in that office. Is that suable?"

"When did it happen?" she asked wearily.

I had the horrible feeling I was doing a Hey-Doc, a family joke about parties at which people would come up to my father and say, "Hey, Doc, I got this pain in my shoulder. What do you think it is?" *I'll make it up to you*, I thought. *I'll read your first novel. I'll buy you lunch.*

"I was fired three years ago."

"That's still in the statute of limitations. You could sue her."

Rachel turned toward Pierrepont Street, and I headed to Gristedes for a carrot cake and ice cream. The fury of my Mastiff Geyser eruption with Alix turned into the continuous simmering of a fumarole. The next three months were hazed by sugar and walking dogs in the heavy-skied days of winter. It felt like every bag of shit I scooped up was talking to me. Not only was I a patsy and a bad agent, I was willfully helpless.

I had justified my passivity in the job by thinking I was on a cliff. Three years later I got it: I wasn't on a cliff; I was against a wall, a solid one built out of the law.

Alix owned the company. What could I do?

Instead of being a puerile asshole, I could have sued her ass, that's what.

I could not live with that piece of myself. So I didn't. I ate and I raged.

"I suggested you sue her when you were working for her," my therapist, the Good Doctor Miller, said.

"You did?" I was shamed further by this. Not only was I willfully ignorant and helpless, I didn't listen to plausible solutions, either.

"You can still sue her," she went on.

I studied the orange tulips on her credenza. If there were tulips to be found on the Upper East Side, she had them. The fresh flowers made her tiny office less of a prison cell of neuroses. "I'm not litigious," I answered at last. "It's another doctor's family thing." This was a point of contention between us.

"Call me if you need me," she would say, and I'd remember Mary, one my father's patients, who'd get liquored up and keep him on the phone for what seemed like hours. I've put up with running out of antidepressants, bad fevers, bronchitis, and getting admitted to the hospital because I didn't want to pull a Mary.

"I'm sorry that I didn't understand how shaken you were by being fired," the Good Doctor Miller repeated. She'd known all along that it was the best thing that could happen to me, a belief I shared intellectually. "But did it ever occur to you that it wasn't because you were so passive, that you never stood up for yourself, that she fired you? Because you did. She pushed you and pushed you, and you finally pushed back. That's how I interpret it. If you'd kept your mouth shut, you'd have had another two or three years there."

Two or three more years? I could feel my toes turning cold.

It could be, of course, that she was right. Alix didn't want a peer in the office. She wanted to be the reigning diva, and brag and storm to a waiting frisson of envy and fear.

When it came to standing up for myself, I was a sentry asleep at the gate.

"All you probably need to do is send her a letter," Doctor Miller said. "She's a bully, Frances. Most bullies will back down when faced with another bully. Wouldn't you enjoy scaring her?" She clapped one hand over her mouth and shook her head. "I didn't say that, did I?"

I like my fluffy-haired, plump shrink best when she is being mildly vindictive.

I didn't sue. I went on eating and raging.

Right up to March 9, when I stepped on the scale and was bitch-slapped with the hundred pounds I'd gained.

In 2002, when I put on my first pair of size 8 trousers, I did not think that I had "graduated," although I described reaching goal weight as the first project I'd ever finished. The problem was, I hadn't come close to finishing myself. Perhaps "initiating" is the better word choice for the blob of self I was left with in the Ann Taylor dressing room.

The problem of the unfinished or unstarted self is that what we once used to compensate for its gaps—food and weight, and then the focused expectation of dieting—is gone, with an unfamiliar body left to absorb the nicks and dings of being alive. That unpadded body and our confusions about it and the new possibilities open to us can, in themselves, cause some of those dings.

"I'm not paying you to shop for clothes!" Alix raged at me one day for a reason I don't remember. Another day she hustled into my office, shut the door behind her, and rushed up to me, stripping off her jacket. "Look at these arms!" she demanded. "Look at them! Do they look like the arms of a fifty-seven-year-old woman?"

Such comments preyed upon the vulnerability I felt in my new body. She would not have said them to me if I weighed 220 pounds or had weighed 150 pounds for a long time. She wouldn't have said them if I hadn't been so vocal about my physical insecurities. Nor would she have said them if I'd told her to cut it the fuck out.

From 1999 to 2003, I'd lived in a normal-sized body, much of that time devoted to learning how to walk and run and dress, reviving my writing life, practicing smiling and speaking less stridently and more quietly. These are all necessary, but I had not acquired the certainty of that ineffable Frances who does not depend on other people's opinions of her to create a self. Both the process of losing weight and the

Stepfords teach one to wait, a good skill in many ways but sometimes a stance that delays necessary actions. Nor had I come into adulthood with a sense of safety or future.

Did I set out to gain weight? Most days, I am one of those women who want to be thin and want to eat. Although I've used laxatives at intervals, I found them more punishing than my disappointed hopes of getting abstinent. I am a failed bulimic.

On the other hand, perhaps I did want to get fat, to brutalize myself beyond the abasement of gobbling and gorging, the hangovers of sugar, the depression and waking shame of being fired and out of control. I may have needed the full monte, food *and* distorting my body, to finish getting rid of the self I had fixed cosmetically but not, adequately, metaphysically. In interfering with my precarious self, Alix and others had done a laughably inadequate job. *I* would show them how it should be done. In this, I am supremely competent.

Two years of working in dangerous unpredictability and being fired, bookended a month before with breaking up with a man I loved and a month after with a man I was terribly fond of, were the triggers of my relapse, but they are neither the causes nor the reasons for it.

The cause of my relapse is most probably written into my DNA. It's certainly grooved into my behavior, and I had arrived at a place in which the stories I'd told myself since childhood, and the stories about myself that I was told, converged so tightly that the sinkholes in my psyche gave way and the only thing I had to fill those caverns with was food.

My dissociation from complex feelings and my difficulty in staking my boundaries make me easy quarry for emotional hyenas, people who thrive on creating uncertainty in those they perceive as weak, throwing off ambiguous directions and changing tactics until their object is dizzy with fear, confusion, or dependence before going in for the kill.

Even well-meaning people confuse me. It's apropos that my insecurities have given rise to a lot of canine references over the years.

"You sound like you were adopted from a pound," my therapist, the Good Doctor Miller, said at least once a month when I moaned about my disbelief that any enterprise would succeed or how difficult it was to foist myself out of the Bat Cave to see a movie.

One of the well-known diet and fitness writers who had blurbed *Passing for Thin*, Pam Peeke, demanded a meeting with me a few months before the book was published. "I loved your book," she said as she expertly gauged my weight. "But I knew you'd gain weight. You're a bit of a lost puppy."

They're right, although the statements, uttered by professionals, codify my infantilism too categorically. I'm susceptible to becoming whatever someone I respect says I am.

Woof.

"Do you want to find your birth mother?" the Good Doctor Miller will go on to ask, just as everyone who finds out I'm adopted asks. "She gave you up, what, forty-some years ago. Isn't it time to go on?"

I shake my head no.

"The people who changed my diapers and got up in the middle of the night because I had nightmares are my parents," I say.

But there is more. The thought of finding the right words to apologize to my birth mother, and the betrayal to the mother and father I have cleaved so fiercely to, make me feel like a sheet of paper torn raggedly in half and then in quarters.

The story I was told was that my parents got a call one night that a baby was available for adoption. They jumped at the chance, scrambling to find bottles from the attic and borrow a crib, reopening Christmas cards to add my name, which they'd picked out years earlier.

It's a lovely story and a true one, as is the story my brother Jim, who was nearly seven years old when I was born, tells of going downstairs to warm the bottle when I woke in the night, relieving Mom of the necessity of getting up.

But of course to the woman who gave birth to me, I was a mistake.

Is there an adopted kid who doesn't know this about him/herself? Whether she wanted me or not is moot. I'd put the poor woman through nine months of fear, discomfort, and, possibly, grief.

I took this pain to confession when I was in graduate school. The priest soothed me by telling me that while *she*, unmarried, was in sin, I, her bastard, was not.[20] This did not assuage my guilt, and I went away more strongly convinced that I had put her through months (and oh, what if it is years?) of misery. It is my oldest guilt, soon followed by my fat. I learned guilt early. I was six years old when I first entered the dark box with my small list of misdemeanors and recited the Confiteor:

> . . . *I have sinned through my own fault,*
> *in my thoughts and in my words,*
> *in what I have done, and in what I have failed to do . . .*

This, too, is part of the story I told myself in whatever formless way a very young child has.

I was a kid with a gothic imagination. I dressed my Barbies up as inmates of the state orphanage in St. Ignatius and, in second grade, after reading a *Reader's Digest* article about throat cancer, was afraid to go to sleep at night because I was sure my parents planned to give me a tracheotomy. Don't even ask what I, age seven, went through after seeing *The Diary of Anne Frank* on a Saturday night when my oldest brother, Dick, was supposed to be babysitting me, or how both my brothers Jim and Dick, seven and nine years older than I, used to hold me down and keep my eyelids open as the Scarecrow, Tin Man, Cowardly Lion, and Toto tried to enter the castle of the Wicked Witch of the West.

These rather picayune anecdotes have several things in common. I was impressionable. Left to myself, I was of a melancholic humor. I

---

20   It was small consolation when a story circulated later that he was removed as chaplain when he made his entrance for Easter Mass dressed as a bunny.

was left to myself a lot and swallowed my aloneness with large doses of food and paranoia.

Why would I think my parents would cut a hole in my throat?

Because out of the witches' brew of being a mistake, I had transmuted to being not only unwanted but unwantable.

"You know no one can stand you, don't you?"

We were downstairs. Dick was racking up the pool balls while I pedaled slowly on the stationary bicycle. He took his opening break shot, and the balls scattered with a loud *tock* followed by a heavy roll. The sound felt a lot like my heart.

"Don't you?" He looked at me over the top of his glasses. "I mean, look at you, Chunky. You're fat. You're ugly. You have no friends. Mom works so much because she can't stand being around you. You're disgusting."

I pedaled a little slower. One of the bright balls cracked in a carom, and Dick swore under his breath.

"That's another thing," he went on. "You have a foul mouth and terrible breath. Do you ever brush your teeth? Shit, I don't think you bathe, you stink so much. It's a wonder anyone can stand you."

I started pedaling backwards on the bike. This was forbidden but I did it anyway. Dick held his pool cue at his side like a scepter, watching me.

"You know this, don't you? Don't you?"

He could pierce steel with those eyes. I was thirteen years old. My mother was rarely around because she was working seventy hours a week bringing the Catholic Church into the 1970s. I sniffed back a gob of snot, hoping to hold back the tears.

"*Don't you?*"

"I . . ." What could I say? I had friends because St. Anthony's was a small school, and I'd known my classmates since kindergarten. But they didn't come over much and everyone seemed to have paired off with a best friend. Terry and Sandy; Wendy and Shannon; Mary Kay and Karen; Patty and Stacy. They were talking about eighth grade and cheerleading, about boys they liked, about the clothes they were amassing for high school, and about the Girl Scout bicycle trip to Minnesota I would not be making.

"I have friends," I said shakily.

"Right," he snorted. He jawed a ball, and I watched it ricochet back and forth as though it were a hypnotist's pocket watch. "Your faggy friend, Jerry. He's not a friend; he's a freak. You can't afford to hang out with freaks."

"Jerry's not a freak," I said in as stout a voice as I could manage.

"He's a freak and so are you. He doesn't love you either, you know. He just likes this big house. Admit it, France. No one can stand you, and no one loves you." I got off the bicycle looking toward my old playroom in the scary, unfinished half of the basement, but I was rooted to the spot. "I'll make a deal with you, okay?" Again with the cold blue eyes, bugging out, it seemed, over his beaky sunburned nose.

"Okay," I said in a tiny voice.

"I will love you."

This was my dream come true! All I'd ever wanted was for Daddy, Dick, and Jerry to love me. Of course I loved many people, but that secret, most painful chamber in my heart didn't include my mother or my brother Jim. They were around so little and had so little interest in me that they were extraneous to this trio of men I would be glad to die for. Daddy, Dick, and Jerry could never love me as fiercely as I loved them, but oh!—if only they loved me a little!

"Okay." My voice was stronger now.

"But here's the deal. You love who I say you love."

I cocked my head. "Huh?"

"You only love who I say you can love."

"You mean, like I ask if it's okay to love Daddy?"

"Right. And you can love Dad." Even Dick, twenty years old with a wife and baby, was too scared of Dad to not love him.

"And Mom?"

"No. Mom is a whore. She's in love with Father Gallagher."

"Liz and Lisa?" His wife and baby daughter.

"Yes. But not Jerry."

I sucked my lips in and bit down. I loved Jerry. I was in love with Jerry. Dick could no more stop that than he could stop daylight from fading to dusk. I had one exception that I kept to myself when I accepted his offer.

"Your mother," my aunt Jane repeated, "doesn't know what love is. If she did, she'd put you on a diet, and she'd stay home and take care of your dad. She doesn't deserve your father."

I was in eighth grade, and my parents were in Hawaii. I was staying with my aunt and uncle and four cousins. Aunt Jane had come into my room, closed the door, and started talking at me. I was sitting on the floor between the bed and the wall, crying.

Sister Theresa had said pretty much the same thing when she pulled me aside to tell me to tell my mother to buy me a slip, that my blouse gapped and my brassiere showed. My Scout leaders also had things to say about my mother's absence and my appearance and sullenness, only they said them when they thought I was asleep. My grandparents and Aunt Mildred were more circumspect in their criticism, but it was there. Mom herself told me that my aunt Claire took her to task for letting me get so fat. One of the most humiliating moments was when Mary Rose Bremmer came up to me at recess and told me I needed to use deodorant. Mary Rose Bremmer! Her family was so poor that the white in the plaid of her uniform was gray, and she brought her peanut butter sandwich and apple lunch in a used paper sack .

But she didn't stink and I did.

It was as though the earth had twisted on its axis. I grew fatter. I had messy periods that required underwear with plastic crotches. I wore my father's shirts with the uniform my mother now made for me with bitter sighing as she hemmed its eight thousand pleats. My old friends spoke a foreign language of pierced ears and wore velvet chokers. I smelled of sweat, and I farted grossly because I went weeks without a bowel movement. My teachers, aunts, grandmother, and classmates confirmed what Dick had spelled out to me. I was as unlovable as I was unwantable.

Or was that the other way around?

It didn't matter. My mother was away from home, and my father lacked the skills for raising a daughter; without my parents' involvement and coaching at the vulnerable age of first loves and first periods, I was ill-prepared for adolescence. That story I'd told myself about being given up, given *away*, was graphically illustrated in my mother's schedule and my helplessness to be like other people.

I stuck to Dick's pact, except for my unrequited love for Jerry, until I was nineteen when, on New Year's Day, Dick skied off to Canada with his preschool-age daughters, disappearing for three months. The spell broke when he broke so many hearts. When he was found, a family council was convened to talk to him about what he had done and not done with his life. I remember that Jim got down on his knees and begged Dick to see the terror and grief he'd caused by abducting Lisa and Jennifer. Dick sat in the swivel easy chair next to the living room doors and stared at Jim like he was a specimen from a freak show, much as he'd pinned me to my inadequate self seven years earlier.

I broke the pact over this, but the spell waned slowly as I learned some grown-up facts. For one thing, Dick was a compulsive liar. He belittled and hit his wives. He would, he told me, "fuck any woman except Mom."

My aunt Jane would die of ammonia on the brain, an alcoholic's disease. Sister Theresa would one day apologize for the way she treated me. "I hated being a nun," she explained, "until my mother died and I could decide for myself if I wanted to be one or not. It turns out I did." Later, too, I would realize that my aunt Claire loved talking to me and was proud of her niece who had gone off to graduate school and a literary career in the East. So, too, I have friends, including Jerry, from St. Anthony's and have forged a close and loving relationship with my parents, who, I've come to understand, have a genius for children under the age of three and over the age of eighteen.

I still obsess over whether my buttons gape.

In college, I found absorption in my studies, and later, in teaching, in publishing, and in writing, for my work. Mom's church friends would become my friends. I would read about sociopathy.

When I graduated from high school, my parents asked me what I wanted. "A car and a shrink," I told them. My first therapist described my parents as having dropped me at his doorstep with a note: "We tried to raise her. You do the rest." We accomplished some big things in our years together. He made me feel my talents were real, and I felt he appreciated me. He downsized my fantasies but didn't suffer me letting go of my dreams of writing. What neither Dr. Michael nor I understood was that as long as I was eating I couldn't grow up. Certainly we recognized that I responded to life by eating—a bad habit or a lack of willpower that resulted in an enormous body that my family and friends could blame my intense moods and lack of boyfriends on.

But I wasn't simply eating instead of living, I learned when I went into the Rooms twenty years later. I was drugging myself so heavily that I couldn't process the typical growing-up stuff of breakups, broken friendships, bad grades, sundry failures, and crushes, learn from it, or move on. In that chemically induced emotional stagnation, I couldn't outgrow being unwanted, unwantable, unloved, unlovable, and on most days, as long as I had food, I didn't really have to recognize those feelings. Nor did I inhabit a body that gave me the confidence, ability, or attractiveness to go through the usual age-appropriate experiences.

My childhood was not *Bleak House*, and this portrait of it doesn't include how my mother made reservations at the English Inn in Victoria so that I could sleep in a canopied bed and booked us for tea at the Empress Hotel, or how my father woke me at midnight to show me the aurora borealis flickering over Flathead Lake. I don't have time to describe Dick driving through snowstorms all night from Seattle to be home for Christmas or Jim dancing a four-year-old me around the ice rink. These are also part of the story, and while I give them miserably short shrift here, they may be precisely what allow me to believe in a grace bestowed on me as much as on any other recovering addict.

Kyrie eleison.

THREE

June

I Believed in the Dream

I began doing interviews for the book in earnest in June. One of the first people to volunteer was Katie, a lurker rather than participator, on my Amazon blog. Her three-time achievement of breaking four hundred pounds and accomplishing two two-hundred-pound losses made me pounce. We talked a few days after she had gone back into OA and gotten abstinent, when she was full of the amazement that comes with getting off the cruise control of bingeing. Getting on a food plan and sticking to it was crucial to her insurance company's requirements for gastric bypass surgery, which she badly wanted to have. She was exhausted from the fight to lose and maintain great amounts of weight, exhausted from eating, exhausted from the limitations of her life.

Saturday became our time to talk that summer and long into the humid limpid nights of Brooklyn I answered her questions about being fat and being thin that were a form of comparing notes. We had a bond in our experiences with twelve-step programs that went a little further than my seedling friendships with the Angry Fat Girls.

Lindsay had never weighed as much as Katie and I did, and neither Mimi nor Wendy had ever gotten as thin as we had. I felt as though Katie's need to talk about fat and thin was a sanity check, while her need to tell stories was an *in*sanity check. I could verify the former but not the latter: I'd done too many stupid things in my thinnitude, and her tales were often too hilarious or too gut-wrenching to certify the teller of them as a candidate for electroconvulsive therapy.

Sometimes I felt she wanted to be that crazy. She would at least be taken care of, with no decisions to worry her.

"New York is magical at Christmas," Phillip kept telling Katie in the two weeks they had known each other. "You've *got* to come with me: I booked this room three months ago."

"That should have been my first clue," she told me during one of our Saturday night conversations. Her voice switched from his salesman technique to a lower octave of sarcasm. "I mean, it was two friggin' weeks before New Year's Eve, and the cluck-head didn't have someone to take to New York? I was such a jerk."

Or naïve. It was 1992 and at twenty-six, Katie was thin for the first time in her life. What experience did she have that would warn her about Phillip?

When they checked into their hotel, she became fascinated by the fact that the only colors in the room were the raffia insets of the closet doors and the oversized print of *Woman in Blue Reading a Letter*. At first Katie felt like a total hipster sitting on the white cotton chair, facing the white bed with the big Vermeer adding another cool touch to the cold starkness of the room. When she and Phillip came back from dinner or looking at the windows of Saks and Lord & Taylor in their Christmas glory, she sat at the desk and studied the painting. She didn't know what irritated her more, Phillip or the *Woman in Blue*.

What was it about the painting that so saddened her? She posited that the woman's obvious pregnancy came first. She wore a long shirt over her skirt, the way Katie wore tunic things for years. The letter didn't make the lady happy, and her pensiveness worried Katie. Was it news that her husband was lost at sea? Katie scratched her head, trying to retrieve what she knew about Holland. Had the woman's mother died of consumption in faraway Emmenthaler, or had her brother's tulip business gone bankrupt in Heinken? Was the baby not her husband's and would he beat her for her infidelity? Was she even married? Was the letter from Hans who had decided to ship off to the New World rather than marry the woman he'd knocked up?

Or did her feeling of unease have nothing to do with the painting? It could have been the "Hello, Jerry" T-shirt complemented by the denim *Seinfeld* baseball cap that Phillip hoovered up in the NBC Store and hadn't changed out of since. Did he *have* to get the cap in denim, for God's sake? Did he have to wear a T-shirt with a fat man on it? Why did he insist on dinner at Tavern on the Green that night? For less money, they could have a better meal at Strip House and she could go shoe shopping before.

The reservations at Tavern on the Green, he informed her, had been made in the same round of phone calls that nailed down the hotel room back in September.

Katie groaned when she heard that and gave a great roll of her eyes. That he didn't notice the expression on her face was another sign because whatever Katie feels is right out there for the world to read.

"You have to understaaand, Fraaances," she said with the elongated flattened vowels of a kid who is inserting an idea of what she wants into her mother's mind rather than coaxing, asking, or arguing for it. "All my friends warned me that traveling with a guy I'd been on four dates with was a baad idea. What did *I* know? He was, like, the second or third guy I'd ever been out with. I mean, I was twenty-six years old! I'd lost 177 pounds and knew as much about dating as a six-year-old. Or a *three*-year-old. By six, kids are counting who goes to whose birthday parties. I was already so chubby in first grade that I wasn't being asked to all the parties."

"So what about Phillip-Hel*lo-Je*rry and New York?" I asked, trying to get her back on topic.

On the morning of the thirtieth, Katie rebelled. He could stand in line to go up to the top of the Empire State Building, but she was taking her 160-pound self up Madison Avenue.

That night, after disappointing him by refusing champagne and taking pictures of him drunkenly posing with topiaries, Katie returned to contemplating the contents of the letter in the painting. Phillip droned on from brochures from lobbies and theater-district restaurants. He had ideas. "Baaad ideas," she inserts. His ideas made them stick out like tourists. They might as well have been wearing those foam Statue of Liberty crowns. Katie hated looking like a tourist. She *hated* it! This getaway that was supposed to be a classic romantic gesture had turned into Phillip's manic search for New York clichés, set off by the sadness of the five-foot painting behind the bed.

He nudged her awake at six on Saturday morning. "Kate, we gotta get moving."

"Wha—?" she mumbled.

"It's New Year's Eve. The *Today* show is definitely gonna have some big star playing. And I wanna take pictures of Times Square."

Katie hauled herself to the bathroom for a quick wash while Phillip made coffee. She pulled on her jeans and the black cashmere sweater she had bought at DKNY the day before, admiring how now that she was thin, she could pull on clothes that were so plain but so gorgeous and she didn't have to say a word about herself. She could run a brush through her ear-length red hair, pinch some color into her cheeks, watch her eyes grow greener under her freshly waxed eyebrows, and look better than when she'd spent an hour getting dressed back in the fat days. She gulped coffee while Phillip got dressed. He would press forward in the crowds outside the NBC studios, wearing his Seinfeld hat, cheering for Mariah Carey or Kris Kross or some damned pop star, as if he cared about that junk back in San Francisco. The woman in blue went on reading with palpable thoughtfulness. Katie decided the woman's mother hadn't died yet but had taken a turn for the worse. She would pack a small trunk and catch a coach bound inland to tend her mother. The baby would be born in the house she had been born in, but the woman in blue would succumb to childbed fever.

"You go ahead," she told Phillip when they got to the excited crowd south of Rockefeller. "I want to look at the Met Store windows."

As soon as he threaded his way in, she walked to the comparative quiet of the angel-lined mezzanine and pulled out her cell phone. It was seven fifteen. She needed two hours. "United?" she said. "I want a flight out of New York to San Francisco as soon after ten this morning as you can book me. I don't have bags to check."

Katie Monahan had a hundred of these tales from her thin days. Her trip with Phillip to New York City for New Year's Eve was my favorite. When Katie was abstinent, as she was that weekend in 1992, she zotted off in every direction at once—dating, making friends, being the life of the party, bringing in good sales, traveling at the drop of her American Express card. Wherever she was, she was dying to belong, and belong at the level of the insider. When she felt outside a group or a city or a family, she felt it in her muscles and nerves

She was, her therapist said, "fluid." At an early holiday party, Phillip laughed until he cried at her stories of the proctologists with whom she visited to talk up her line sulfasalazine and 5-ASA drugs, then came on like gangbusters with invitations for drinks and movies and, finally, the suggestion they go to New York. She went along with it because . . . well, he seemed to like her and she'd never had a real boyfriend and her mother had harped on her throughout her adolescence that she'd never get a husband if she were fat. With Phillip, she didn't have to do anything. He took care of where they went on their dates, where they ate, drank, and made out. The phone calls and invitations were exciting, as was dressing up for dates and planning what to take and what to do in New York. It was easy to go with the flow.

In that Christmas week, the four-hundred-year-old image of a sad woman and Phillip's making her look at every picture he took of the topiary at Tavern on the Green brought on a fit of melancholy that demanded some kind of big action. Clearly, Phillip was a loser. So she dumped him without so much as leaving a note in their hotel room.

And anyway, the sex was . . . odd. Or she was odd while having sex. She kept thinking of Annie Hall getting out of bed to sketch while she and Alvy made love. Part of her was sitting in that white chair, considering the painting, studying *Zagat* and *New York Magazine* for what would provide the best stories back home.

Katie loves Christmas, but it has never been kind to her.

Katie had read my Amazon blog about my relapse when she wrote me in May, volunteering to be interviewed for this book. I was intrigued by her history. At the age of twenty-six, she weighed 160 pounds after losing 177 pounds. She maintained that weight for a year. A decade later, she went from 400 pounds to 140 pounds for a year, then topped 400 pounds. I was impressed that she could gain 287 pounds in four years. Clearly, this was a woman of grit and determination.

We needed few preliminaries. The first thing we agreed upon was that the first ingredient of relapse is the cold-water shock of success. The second thing we understood about our relapses was that the Rooms where we got thin contributed to them.

Katie and I had had similar, but not identical, food plans. The general difference was that she had fewer whole carbohydrates than I, but we both, when we were in the Rooms, weighed and measured our food and we abstained from sugar and flour. Her first weight loss, at twenty-six, occurred under the aegis of Overeaters Anonymous, and her second, ten years later, happened while she was in FA, Food Addicts in Recovery Anonymous.[21]

---

21 OA (Overeaters Anonymous) is the acronym for one of a number of twelve-step-based programs for recovery from eating disorders. Others include ABA (Anorexics and Bulimics Anonymous), CEA-How (Compulsive Eaters Anonymous—Honest, Open-minded and Willing to listen), EAA (Eating Addictions Anonymous), EDA (Eating

FA is a very strict program in which everyone follows the same food plan and works the steps in closed groups with a checklist of behaviors one cannot engage in. They are the Jets in the gangland of eating disorder groups. Organized, insular, perhaps rightfully bragging about what they do, FAers tend to socialize among themselves. "They were the cool ones," Katie, the perpetual wannabe insider, said. "I felt like I really belonged when I was in FA."

She got really thin in FA. The pictures of her at 140 pounds showed a woman with many angles—collarbones and shoulder blades, high cheekbones and the thin woman's smile that peels back the flesh around the mouth more than the fat woman's smile. And her smile was brilliant.

For all that Katie felt like one of the Heathers in FA, she was never good enough for its rules. One of those rules was to reach the MetLife weight goal. Katie is five feet five inches tall and was expected to lose another fifteen pounds. "At 140, I was sickly and cold and miserable and hungry all the time. I asked for my food plan to be adjusted but it was another case of 'You just want more food because you don't have any willingness.'"

Willingness is one of the key words in twelve-step programs. Be willing to go to a meeting. Be willing to read *Voices of Recovery* or work on your fourth step. Be willing to put a behavior down for one day or a half hour. Be willing to take direction.

Direction was one of Katie's stumbling blocks. Sponsors insisted on synchronizing watches and calling (at five a.m. in her case) on the dot. Call a minute late, and she'd hear she was "taking her will back," which is the opposite of willingness.

In the end, she said, "It's a fucking cult. I couldn't join the step

---

Disorders Anonymous), FAA (Food Addicts Anonymous), FA (Food Addicts in Recovery Anonymous), GSA (Grey Sheeters Anonymous), RA (Recoveries Anonymous), and RFA (Recovering from Food Addiction).

studies because I smoked and drank Diet Coke. You can't take anti-depressants, and I was never thin enough for them. You're either with them or not, and no matter how much weight I lost, there was always something wrong about me."

After two years of FA, in 2002, the gang mentality had stripped Katie of her fragile sense that she was good enough to belong, pushing her into another of her notorious depressions. She went back to her beloved cakes, feeling bleak and without faith, "like sitting in a dark room with a lead jacket—the one they put on you at the dentist for X-rays—and the room just keeps getting smaller and I just keep getting bigger."

Worsening her depression were the teachings of the Rooms, which can throw a lot of blame on the addict. Her FA group was intolerant of relapse—consider the browbeating being a minute late for a phone call engendered, and you'll have an idea of how backs turn for breaking abstinence. I had an acquaintance in FAA, another very strict recover group, who lost her day count over using a tablespoon of the wrong soy sauce.[22]

"It's a criminal act to be fat or 'in the food' or 'struggling with the food,'" Katie blogged on her own site, Mrs. Beasley Says So. She was frozen out of the group. To admit to an outright binge risks losing one's sponsor and being shunned by other members. They're more frightened of the same thing happening to them than they are sympathetic to relapse. Speaking as a serial relapser myself, one becomes wary of consistently burdening a group with the announcement of three days or twenty-seven days of adherence to a food plan, or the redundant plaint of being unable to get abstinent. That self-consciousness itself can drive those most in trouble away.

---

22   Rather than emphasizing calories consumed or pounds lost, all eating disorder twelve-step groups recognize and reward the number of back-to-back days of adhering to the individual's food plan.

Relapse along with weight gain was the worst crime Katie could commit. "My friends in that program, and myself included, have had to hate fat," she added. How could "recovery" from compulsive eating occur when, through group-think, you turned your back on what you have been most of your life? It encouraged self-hatred, and Katie always lived on that edge. Three years of bingeing, crying, therapy, and raging later, Katie warned others, "Don't hate yourself into weight loss. It won't work, it won't last, and please love yourself into acceptance. Don't be afraid of Fat Acceptance. Embrace it and don't deny who you are."

I must interject that not all recovery programs, or all FA groups, encourage such fat phobia among its members. The Stepfords have always taught me and others to thank God for our fat, which was very possibly a life-saving, albeit inadequate, reaction to situations we couldn't otherwise have borne.

At the same time, how many relapses come from losing a lot of weight—enough to shop in misses' departments and be asked out on streams of dates—but not enough or, in some cases, an uncomfortable amount of weight?

In her first weight loss, when Katie reached 160 pounds, she was thin enough for economy class, designer clothes, and boyfriends, but when she got to 160 pounds, a size 10, a decade later, a group of women who had never been weighed on a loading dock scale deemed her still fat.

The more Katie lost, the more bewildered she was by the choices, possibilities, abilities, and changed dynamics with her colleagues, family, and friends. Black boatneck sweater or ivory muslin blouse? Should I change jobs or go after a promotion? What do I do with all this energy? The gauntlet of classic exchanges that are both flattering and insulting become wearying. "I remember standing to meet an old friend I'd been out of touch with for years" Katie said of her FA weight loss. Her friend's eyes widened and Katie said, "This is what I really look like." Her friend leaned in to kiss her and said, "I always thought you were beautiful."

"What *bullshit!*" I spat. "I mean, you *are* beautiful, but if she'd always thought so, why wasn't she setting you up on dates or asking you out with a male friend as your partner? Why wasn't she asking you to go to Mexico with her or clothes shopping?"

"Yup," she said. "Beautiful and fat and left out."

The more she fit in with the anonymous crowds waiting for BART in the morning, the more exposed and, ultimately, fraudulent Katie felt among people she knew.

The dream that Katie bought into is that losing weight will make us beautiful, reverse the clock, get us the marvelous life we have watched other people having. But we are unprepared for living naturally in our now-thin bodies, which, as Katie experienced in her second weight loss through Food Addicts Anonymous, are not always good enough.

Fed up (pun intended) with the rigors and philosophies Katie couldn't meet or embrace, she found it easy to skip a meeting, drift away from her sponsor, go into a bakery and get a dozen of anything. One of the few joys, in fact, of relapse is not, for twenty pounds or so, getting dirty looks for buying a pint of ice cream and eating it on the street.

Crawling, three or more hundred pounds crushing her knees, into the Rooms, and getting abstinent on a strict and highly exclusionary food plan is a setup for bingeing. All it takes is one slipup. In the Rooms, people warn themselves of how powerful cravings and dependency become once they've been indulged by saying, "My disease isn't asleep. It's doing push-ups."

Years of watching everyone else enjoy birthday cake and Thanksgiving stuffing, years of Saturday nights without popcorn or pizza, weddings and showers attended without a drop of champagne and having to ask the cater-waiters what's in the salad dressing: abstinence makes us outsiders as much, in ways, as our obesity did.

There is a lot of catching up to do.

In relapse, we still continue to have the hope of finding peace with food in the Rooms, so why not eat the grand slam? We know our fat asses will be back in uncomfortable folding chairs as we cross our arms protectively across our chests and keep our heads down in the shame of having fucked up.

What was recently our best friend—the community of fellow overeaters—fades and we return to what helped us survive for so long. "Ice cream is my lover," one blog reader wrote me, and another, watching the nubile students from NYU walking through the long dusks of June, sighed, "I went to OA for a while, but picked up more craziness and self-absorption there than I had before."

"It really is a miracle that I went back to regular OA," Katie said of her latest reentry, that June of 2006. "In FA, I lost faith in anything Higher Power–like."

I disagree with her notion that there was a miracle involved. Katie had tried Weight Watchers and every diet on Amazon and the magazine racks: How could she not go back to the only thing that had worked for her? She wanted gastric bypass, but having surgery was contingent upon losing some weight and its success would depend on her sticking to a strict food plan. The Rooms were her only alternative, whether she took God in with her or not, and she needed a sponsor who didn't try to become a Higher Power by smacking her hands with a ruler for calling at 5:04 a.m.

The first thing you have to understand about Katie is that she had what could be called emotional fibromyalgia. A car backfiring could make her furious (*Why doesn't that idiot take his car into the shop— people are trying to work here!*), jealous (*Lucky guy—he has the money to get it fixed.*), despairing (*My car is going to die anytime.*), or go off on a wild tangent that could consume days of research and fantasizing (*I'm moving to Venice, where there are no cars and no rules against smoking.*).

An annoyance someone else would laugh off in the course of a day could send her spinning for a week. The cause of the annoyance was often of her own making, which she acknowledged and then heaped more blame on herself for. There was that company meeting she had attended, in which she categorically laid out what their training program was lacking. She wasn't lambasting the person in charge of training new salespeople, but she was clear about what wasn't working. I might have couched such criticism by softening it with "my experience and the latest research suggests" or "other companies are finding success by," but Katie jumped in with salient, imperative points. Her boss was pleased: a successful salesperson with a degree in organizational behavior brings a lot to these bimonthly summit councils. The training manager got into a major snit that, of course, got back to Katie.

"I'm gonna quit my job," she snarled. "Bunch of assholes. She called me a queen bee. I'm not a queen bee. Am I a queen bee? I wasn't exactly *mean*. I want to see this company expand, and she's not doing her job. Does that make me a queen bee?"

That fluidity her therapist speaks of was in full play. The day after she told me the story, she changed her Gmail icon to a scowling little girl with the words "*I'm* the queen bee around here." Five days after the meeting, she changed the picture to a hive with the caption "There can only be one queen bee."

Katie didn't let go easily.

She was a Gordian knot of sadness, despair, self-loathing, sarcasm, bluntness, anger, gratitude, appreciation, contempt, honesty, and game-playing, each in equal proportion *all the time*. Her therapist had a lot of experience working with borderline personalities and Katie was glad about that because she saw herself in many of the DSM-IV-TR—the revised fourth edition of the Diagnostic and Statistical Manual of Mental Disorders—criteria for the disorder.[23]

---

23 According to the National Institute of Health, "A person with BPD may experience intense bouts of anger, depression, and anxiety that may last only hours, or at most a day. These may be associated with episodes of impulsive aggression, self-injury, and drug or alcohol abuse. Distortions in cognition and sense of self can lead to frequent changes in long-term goals, career plans, jobs, friendships, gender identity, and values."

The good news about having borderline personality disorder is that the condition usually stabilizes after ten years or so.

The bad news about having borderline personality disorder is that, for Katie, it had gone on for more than forty years.

Above all, Katie was full of longing—the way a stray dog longs for scraps or an orphan for a parent—for friends, for her family's acceptance, to be in less pain, to belong, to fit in. One of the reasons that we became friends was because the opportunities she (often unknowingly) gave me to fulfill some of those longings were so blatantly obvious. Wanting love, after all, is coequal to wanting to give it. Katie granted me that supreme pleasure.

Like so many of us, Katie pinned her future on thinness. "I believed in the dream that when I lost weight everything in the world would be better." The one part of her longing that was fulfilled by losing weight was that she fit. Airplane seats and clothes and all those scary moments that we feel so acutely excluded from became available, and Katie embraced them. She who had never traveled much went to Hawaii, the Caribbean, Mexico. "I was able to go anywhere and do anything. I didn't have to think about my clothes or packing . . . everything looked good. I could be having a bad hair day, no makeup, and still feel good." She took yoga, which she loved and missed, she left her clerical job in the district attorney's office and went into sales and made a lot of money. She got a tummy tuck.

It looked to everyone to be the happy ending after years of sad stories, but her success became another aspect of herself that she mourned. "Deep inside I was so sad. I cried all the time. People would say to me, 'What is wrong with you? You're thin! You should be happy!' I believed these comments, and I felt even worse for feeling so bad. Something was terribly wrong with me, and I couldn't figure it out. I became even more self-loathing, and the only soother that has ever made me feel safe was to eat a lot of cake."

We should mandate that all weight-loss compliments be accompanied by, "You have always deserved your thinness," or quote Pam

Peeke's formula, "For every twenty-five pounds removed, it takes one year to mentally adjust. So be kind to yourself, okay?"

Peeke's formula is breathtaking for women like Katie, Wendy, Mimi, and me, who come from very high weights. It means that when Katie was twenty-six, 160 pounds, and a brand-new size 10 after sixteen months of her restricted OA food plan and a loss of 197 pounds, mentally she weighed about 303 pounds. She had the same insecurities of the fat woman who sabotages herself in order to spin her failures, which may explain why she carried a snotty attitude into the workplace and was either fired or quit before she could be fired. A 303-pound woman doesn't *deserve* to make good money, a 303-pound woman has to strike before the name-calling and judgmental looks flatten her, a 303-pound woman doesn't have choices when it comes to men and so will go to New York in order to take an idiot's picture with King Kong carved from privet in a sleet storm outside Tavern on the Green—even though she was a size 10.

Nor would she have collected the experience to understand what healthier, metaphorically broader people learn as they go along. The most important of these lessons is that *it's not about you*—"it" being bad behavior or having emotionally frozen parents, the lack of a man's follow-up after a date. When you're fat, everything is about your fat and, by extension, everything is about you.

"It was almost like being in another world," she said of her last and biggest weight loss. "I was never comfortable; I felt like an imposter." One of her terrors was that new people in her life would find out she had weighed 330 pounds in her recent past. "I really tried to hide the fact that I had ever been fat. Then people who had known me before would say, 'You look so good,' and I thought to myself, 'Yeah, but I should have never been fat in the first place, so it's really not an accomplishment.'"

I wager that every woman who has lost an altering amount of weight has a silent comeback to those compliments. Mine was, "What was I before? Chopped liver?" Mimi had slightly more negative reactions, vacillating between, "What did I look like before?" and "No, I don't. You're just saying that to be nice." Our unspoken responses are as undermining as our low expectations because we reaffirm for ourselves how unacceptable and loathsome our big bodies, and with those bodies, our selves are.

Using Pam Peeke's formula of a year of adjustment for every twenty-five pounds lost, it can take a decade to separate social judgments from our obesity, our obesity and fates from something bad in us, and realize that, like everyone else, our faults and compulsions do not detract from our worthiness as human beings.

In June 2006, as Katie started a new food plan, she avoided meeting with her sponsor as much as possible. She had been on disability, because of her weight and depression, for two months, and she was filling her days with cruising the Internet and becoming absorbed into a reality television series I'd never heard of. For a small fee, she was able to access twenty-four-hour live feeds from the house in which *Big Brother* was being shot, and her sarcasm and incisiveness made her a star in the program chat rooms.

Then it unraveled.

"One of the 'houseguests,'" she emailed me on another of what I had come to think of as our Loser Fat Girl Saturday Nights, "said 'If anybody is on the Internet right now watching this, they are pathetic.' That really affected me. I tried to chat about it with people in the room but they were assholes and just said, I shouldn't let someone I don't know affect how I feel. I started crying really hard."

I called immediately. Although it was impossible to change Katie's mind or feelings, she was, as I said, easy to communicate love to.

"What is the name of the emotion you're feeling over this comment?" I asked.

"Pathetic," she sniffed. "I think being this big and being abstinent is a very strange experience. I feel good about myself because I have made the choice to live and be abstinent, but in the grand scheme of life I feel pathetic."

"It's perfectly okay to feel pathetic," I said. "Just because it's a word we throw out in insults doesn't drain it of its force and honesty when you're in it."

I thought for a moment about what she was going through, barely able to get around, using a stool in her shower because she couldn't stand that long, her public life a series of OA meetings, DBT classes, and therapy. She was going to the hospital to see her gynecologist soon and would have a chance to weigh herself after a couple of weeks of abstinence. She was worried that she hadn't lost weight, and she was humiliated because she had to go to the loading dock to use the scale. Everything Katie did out of the house was a reminder of how disarranged she was. She had a minimal social life for distraction. One friend was moving away, another had a reputation among Katie's friends and family as being a histrionic bitch, and she worried about depending too much on her best friend, Ingrid, who had helped hold her together in the last three years.

"You know how they say in the Rooms that we're only as old as our abstinence?" I asked. The snippets of twelve-step wisdom drove us up a wall, but we spoke the same language from the same context and it provided a shorthand between us.

"You're three weeks old, according to that line of thinking. A three-week-old baby would be doing a lot of crying and depending on other people to take care of her. Add that to the years of abstinence you've had in the past, and you're just about the age where Mom parks you in front of the TV so she can take a shower or clean the kitchen. You're parked in front of the TV. You're on track."

One of the things I loved about talking to Katie is hearing how wise I am . . . and then later having to admit that just about everything she's feeling, I am feeling, too, and, too often, trying not to feel it by eating. In many ways, she was the stronger of us—she at least owned her feelings.

"But Fraaances! It *is* pathetic to be watching a feed at four in the morning and pathetic that it hurts me," she protested.

"Feeling pathetic doesn't mean you *are* pathetic," I said. "This is a cutthroat show, right? They're all trying to be nice *and* get somebody else kicked off. In effect, they're hyenas, looking for the weakest member in a herd of gazelles. These are not nice people. You—and a kazillion other viewers—were dissed by a hyena."

Earlier that spring, in an Amazon discussion of the comments women get for being fat or losing weight, Lindsay observed that "Nobody who gets thin gets rid of their problems, they just trade them in." The only part she got wrong is that we trade in a few problems (like airplane seats), keep the oldest ones (why we got fat, how being fat has shaped our psyches), and receive a handful of new ones in return.

When Lindsay was at her lowest weight in college and working as a waitress at a local restaurant, she hated the attention she got from her fellow waitstaff for her butt. Someone more daring would have wanted the attention, dressed for it, and used it, but Lindsay found it embarrassing. The butt, after all, is a sexual zone. Many Fat Girls have narrow parameters of how much of their sexual selves they will show. Weight loss unwittingly changes those parameters, and we lose a sense of control over how much of ourselves we show and what it means.

If I wear a piece of clothing I consider risky, I'll add another item that is deeply conservative. A camisole will thus be topped by a linen jacket, a short skirt with tights and boys' shoes. It's a formula I've worked out over the years since being thin that still works—one of the biggest lessons I've learned from regaining weight is that I'm still sexual and still seen sexually by some, not entirely insane, people.

Mimi was a graduate student when she was at her thinnest. Studious by nature and informed by her parents that she had to get a degree that would enable her to support herself, she hadn't noticed the college party scene when she was an undergraduate at Duke. "I didn't know how to dress or talk to people," she remembered of that first, most successful weight loss. "Everybody was pairing off and getting married, and I didn't even know how to flirt." Ill-prepared for graduate school comradeship, she slipped back to the company and comfort of food. Is it easier to settle into our new bodies if we've closely observed normies—friends or siblings—over the course of adolescence and young adulthood? Mimi didn't have that growing up and she didn't know how to adapt to her thinness.

One of my blog readers and fellow bloggers, Lia, suggested that her obesity was an escape from sex. A beautiful former model, Lia was in her forties, happily married, happily employed. She also had an advanced degree in psychotherapy, so her context was Freudian. "Sex becomes significant around the Oedipal stage, at five or six. If you're traumatized at that age, the impulse toward sex is a giant threat and you'll do anything you can to block it. When I was eleven, I went from 80 pounds to 120 pounds in six months. My parents said, 'No man will ever want you.' That was great news to me: they just gave me the key to keeping men off me. But the truth is, fat doesn't prevent you from being the object of sexual interest, it only makes you think you're excluded."

Fat as a chastity belt is a possibility that pertains to us all, and to Katie's second relapse in particular. "I had problems dressing vixen-like," she said. "I seemed to go for very middle-of-the-road clothes, with a hint of style. I somehow feel embarrassed to look sexy or to even feel sexy. It's almost like I don't have a right to have sex, be sexy, want sex, or look sexy. This feeling is deep in the caverns of my being. It began long ago."

Identifying with stories told by men in OA or thinking she could save them from their pain, imagining scenes of voluminous salad making with *The Big Chill* soundtrack in the background, she had crushes on guys in recovery, which was a horrible idea. It's easier for men to lose and maintain weight, which can result in competitiveness or inferiority: you're always watching what the other person is ingesting and, newly liberated from their own prisons, the issues around fat, food, and eating are complicated by two sets of neuroses.

Katie's first relapse, in 1993, which resulted in a gain of 270 pounds, had its seeds in a housewarming on her twenty-fifth birthday. Her friend Ingrid raved about the house they were going to, a mansion on Russian Hill owned by the chief of psychiatry at the hospital where Ingrid had her therapy practice. Katie had badly not wanted to spend her birthday alone, and although she wouldn't know anyone but Ingrid at the party, it was better than a night alone in front of the television.

Their host was welcoming, and the two women saw immediately that he'd gone to great lengths to create a stylish affair—the food, music, and décor reflected his Turkish heritage. "I'm so glad Ingrid brought such a lovely friend," he gushed. "My husband and I are delighted to have you celebrate our new home."

There was live music played on strange instruments—a long-necked guitarlike thing, a violin that looked like a fence picket. The food was plentiful and "clean"—that is, on Katie's food plan. She had an Urfa kebob, garlicky and spicy with peppers she had never seen before, and onion salad, and a yogurt drink lightened by cucumber juice. As the raki flowed, the Turkish guests began to dance, inviting their hosts and other males into the circle, and then the younger women.

That is how Katie met Ahmed, the man gripping her right shoulder and laughing as she tried to get the hop-kick step and kicked him in the shin instead. When the dance was over, he disappeared, and Katie looked for Ingrid, who had been given a big red napkin to wave at the end of the chorus line. She ended up on the floor, laughing herself silly and still waving the napkin. As she told Katie what had happened, Katie's dance partner appeared with a glass of club soda with lime and a plate of baklava.

"I am Ahmed. You must eat this. You will be famished from all the dancing we are going to do."

Katie didn't have the baklava, but she danced with Ahmed and Ingrid again and again, some dances involving clenched hands and heavy elbow choreography, some where people hopped and kicked their way in and out of a circle.

"That dance," Ahmed told her, "is usually danced by couples. Some of these dances are for men only. But it's a party!" He smiled, and his face lit up, his warm eyes glittering like the Bay Bridge they could see from the second-floor deck. The trio of musicians had packed up for the night and were having dinner and Dar, Ingrid's boss, had put on the old romantic songs Katie loved.

If Ella Fitzgerald singing "Do I Love You?" hadn't segued into Frank Sinatra's "All the Things You Are," Katie might not have accepted Ahmed's offer of coffee. Blame it on a lyric. Frankie wasn't enumerating anything Katie could use against herself. Anyone could be springtime or the quiet of sunset.

They went to a Starbucks and talked about her work for the DA and the flatlands of Sacramento, where she grew up. He described his roommates, newlyweds who had just emigrated, and where he had grown up, in the hills above the Gulf of Antalya. He asked her to dinner the next night, and she said yes, driving home still burbling with laughter at such an odd night.

"He's persistent, isn't he?" Ingrid asked a week later. Katie had been to dinner with Ahmed on four out of the last seven nights. They'd taken a Saturday drive to Big Sur, and he'd shown her the insider's version of the Tenderloin. That morning, he had sent her a dozen of the tallest yellow roses she'd ever seen, which is when she called Ingrid.

"He's interesting," Katie said. "It's like we're tourists in each other's world."

"Yellow roses, huh? I wonder what *that* means in Turkish . . ."

Katie liked Ahmed. His English was good enough that they could go to the movies and watch TV, his tutorials in the vernacular. Katie is fanatical about pop culture. He cracked her up when she took his hand as they walked down the street, and he said, "Hallelujah, I've died and gone to Kentucky!" or when she told him she liked her steaks rare, "You are alive when they start to eat you. Try to show a little respect."

She felt like she'd been through a meat grinder after spending an evening trying to explain that Maggie Simpson had yet to speak more than one word. It ended with Ahmed shaking his head and saying, "Tell me again, is Bart really a boy?" She buried her head in her hands and moaned until he wrapped her in a big bear hug and whispered into her ear, "I did the whistling belly-button trick at the high school talent show."

Katie's loneliness and tendency to overreact were calmed by Ahmed. In large part, it was due to his limited grasp of English and the trouble he sometimes had communicating. When it comes to her emotional issues, Katie has trouble communicating, too. Ask Katie what she is ashamed of and she will maunder a bit about her high state of emotions and how she gets blamed when her family starts another feud. She will quickly dribble out of reasons. "I dunno. It's all fucked up." Ahmed reacted to her tears by holding her and soothing her, but he didn't often probe into why she was crying.

She felt, with him, that she had escaped living under a microscope.

Three months after they met, Katie moved in with him.

Did she believe he was "Mr. Right"?

No. But it was thrilling to be told she was beautiful, sexy, a wonderful lover. It's thrilling to be able to make someone laugh. It's also another Fat Thing: this man likes me. I have to keep him because no one is ever going to like me this way again.

Soon after she moved in, they made a trip to Bakersfield to introduce him to her family. They stopped for sodas along the way and, as they stretched their legs a bit in a McDonald's parking lot, she said, "My parents and my brother are going to wonder what's up. I don't introduce them to friends very often."

"You can tell them I love you very much," he said firmly.

"*That's* going to lead to a *lot* more questions."

"What do you mean?"

"Like, are you thinking of getting married?"

"Are we?"

Katie put her Diet Coke on the trunk of her car and crossed her arms. "Are we?"

"I love you very much," he said. He smiled slyly. "I want Cowboy George. I don't want no English glitter prince."

Her stepfather and brother froze when Ahmed walked into the living room behind Katie. Ahmed told them he worked in his cousin's luggage shop on Fisherman's Wharf, and Frank Stannert, her stepfather, got up from his easy chair and left the room, shutting the door of his study without saying a word. Her brother Stephen had to put his hand to his mouth to wipe away the sardonic grin that threatened.

"Good money in, uh, suitcases?" Stephen asked.

"We sell souvenirs, too," Ahmed answered. "And all kinds of bags. Pocketbooks, backpacks, wallets—you name it." His voice was defensive, and his black eyes were a piercing stare. "And yes, I have employment authorization. I am legal."

"This is another phase of yours, isn't it?" her mother asked as they did the dishes. "I suppose you're going to convert to Moslem and take Arabic classes. Then you'll be on to—what? Dating a black man? Deciding to move to . . . oh," she grunted more in anger than frustration, "Iceland?"

"First of all, that's not very nice," Katie said. "Second, 'Moslem' is a person who practices Islam. Ahmed is actually a Methodist."

Her mother sighed. "Every time we see you, you're someone new or something different."

Yeah, Katie thought. *Almost two hundred pounds different.* At first everyone was supportive of her weight loss, but when she told them about OA, they rolled their eyes and chalked it up to what she thought of as the family's "Katie Bulletin Board," where they kept track and kept score of her mistakes, moods, tangents, and U-turns. She walked away as she dried the pots and pans, not wanting her mother to see her crying.

Her mother turned off the faucet and threw the sponge down. "I have a headache," she announced. "I'm going to go lie down. You and Ali let yourselves out, won't you? And don't disturb Frank."

Rule # 1 in the Stannert house: Never upset the stepfather.

Rule # 2 in the Stannert house: Never expect anything.

Rule # 3 in the Stannert house: Never say anything important.

Katie liked how Ahmed seemed to absorb her nervousness. She relaxed as he smoked between courses and took his time over the thick coffee he drank; she relaxed more when he had to process a sentence or an event from Turkish to English to American. Whatever it was, he slowed Katie down in a way she hadn't experienced since eating her last pie. "I was full of jittery nervousness," she recalls of being thin. It's a common reaction to the metamorphosis, especially when the former Fat Girl has missed out on normal experiences or been schooled, as Katie had been by her mother, in the dogma that "Nobody is going to hire you if you're fat. Nobody will want to date you if you're fat." She'd gotten thin, and her family still regarded her as a burden. Katie had hoped losing weight would knit her into the family fabric. If she could keep the right job and date a guy who sent yellow roses, would *that* prove to her mom that she was no longer the problem, that she was, in fact, a success? "My disappointment was on the cellular level, and I was like, 'oh shit, this isn't the answer either.'"

Nonetheless, she called her mother a couple of weeks later and told her she was getting married in October. She expected a long silence, and she got it.

"You don't expect us to pay for the wedding, do you?"

"No, Mom, I just want you to come and try to get to know Ahmed. He's not so bad."

"'Not. So. Bad.'" There was another long silence. "Girls in love don't say their fiancé is not so bad. They say 'he's really wonderful when you get to know him.'" Another long silence. "I don't want to upset Frank with all of this. Stephen could come to your wedding, or your grandma and Aunt Sharon."

Stephen wouldn't stop laughing when she called with the news. When she called Michael, her brother in Albuquerque, he sang a little ditty that started, "Marry an A-rab/and you'll drive a-cab . . ."

The rest of the family took the news without insulting her. Grandma Monahan and Aunt Sharon were thrilled at the prospect of planning a wedding.

"What about the Swedenborgian Church?" Aunt Sharon suggested immediately. "It's so intimate and homey."

"I want Sharon to take pictures of you trying on gowns so I can help you decide," Grandma said.

Sharon's husband, Uncle Carl, a detective with the San Francisco Police Department, moaned when Sharon gave him the news. "Get his last name," he said. "I'll check him out."

It hurt Katie's feelings a little, but at least Carl was on her side. At least he, Sharon, and Grandma were *doing* things for her rather than refusing to face the situation.

"What does this 'devil and the deep blue sea' mean?" Ahmed asked.

Katie was stumped for more than a cursory explanation. "I mean, I want my mom and brothers to come but I don't want a guest list and cocktail napkins with our initials on them."

"Let's go to city hall," he said. "That's what Yusef and Ruuya did."

"Grandma and Aunt Sharon would insist on coming, and they'd be all weepy and shaking their heads about not being in a chapel."

"Then we'll go away."

They opted for a sneak-away wedding, with Ingrid as maid of honor, along with Ahmed's cousin, Ammar, as best man and second witness. Katie bought a white bolero suit and stood in the Bloomingdale's dressing room crying. The sleeveless dress showed off her legs and arms, of which she was rightly proud, and the jacket, with its white satin loops along the hem and sleeves, was beautiful. It was a size 10. She was getting married to a man who loved her but came from a culture she knew nothing about. Ingrid kept warning her that she thought they should wait. Her brothers wouldn't be there, and her mother had written her saying she thought it best for the time being that they confine their correspondence to emails and letters. She cried as she walked around the shoe department in her one-hundred-dollar sandals, and she cried as she drove to the small house they had rented in South San Francisco.

The crying jag lasted through the remaining week before the wedding. She was forced to take another couple of days off from work because she couldn't stop, and when, intermittently, she did stop, her face was as puffy and mottled red as a strawberry.

"Kate," Ingrid said as she watched her friend throw things into the overnight bag she was taking to Lake Tahoe. Katie snatched a flannel nightgown and three pairs of underwear and stuffed them in. There was hair conditioner waiting to be packed but no shampoo, all the makeup, Ingrid suspected, Katie had ever owned, red shorts, and an "I ♥ Vegas" T-shirt. "Kate. You can*not* take a flannel nightgown that you wore when you weighed three hundred pounds on your honeymoon. You need sneakers and shampoo. What you really need is to cancel this thing until you're sorted out."

"No," Katie said, pulling out the nightgown, and with it all the clothes tangled in it. She sniffed and clenched her hands, but tears rolled down her face anyway. "I said yes. I do what I say I'll do. But I want my mother," she wailed. "It doesn't feel right that Mom, Stephen, and Michael have refused to come. They haven't even sent cards!"

"Ahmed would understand if you said you wanted to wait until your family is more accepting."

"No, he wouldn't. He asks me every day if I love him, if I'll be his wife. He'd be . . ." She couldn't think of the right word. Heartbroken? Devastated? Somewhere between devastated and very disappointed. "He'd think I'm the sort of person to go back on my word."

Ingrid poured about a quart of foundation and a half pound of powder on Katie, caked on some blush, fluffed her red hair, and drove her from the hotel to the courthouse. If it wasn't for her cadaverish face, Katie would have looked stunning.

Ingrid was dismayed to see that no one brought flowers. When it came time to exchange rings, Katie was ready with a gold band for

Ahmed, but he didn't have one for Katie. He laughed in embarrassment, and Ingrid slid her amethyst pinkie ring off and palmed it over. The I-dos were said, everyone signed the register and walked out into the late afternoon sunlight of a resort town between tourist seasons.

"I am taking Ingrid back to San Francisco, correct?" Ammar asked. Everyone nodded. "I have to work tomorrow and would like to get going."

Ingrid leaned over and kissed Katie. "You're a beautiful bride. Remember: we're married now."

Katie hugged her back, as hard as she could. She could feel sobs rising in her chest, and the deep swallows of tears in her throat. "Thank you," she whispered. "I love you *so* much."

Katie and Ahmed went out for a fancy dinner. She ate more steak than she normally would have but left enough to warrant a doggie bag that came back in tinfoil the waiter had curled into a swan. The swan was the most weddinglike thing about the whole day.

"I want to call my parents," Ahmed said, looking at his watch. It would be seven in the morning in the little town not far from Akseki, which he pointed out on a map. "And my brother. They're waiting to hear that we're married."

Katie felt a pang at that, but also a shadow of what Uncle Carl had warned her of when his investigations didn't turn up heroin trafficking or a criminal record back in Turkey. "These guys—not well-educated, no profession, not here to go to school and better themselves in ways that will contribute to society—these guys often look for vulnerable women to marry in order to get their green card, Katie-Kat. Are you sure he loves you?"

Was he calling for congratulations on finding the woman of his dreams or for his dreams of becoming an American?

"I think I'll take a walk," she said.

"Good idea," Ahmed answered. "This might take a while. And get us something for breakfast while you're out."

The pillow on his side of the bed was rumpled when she came

back. The light was on in the bathroom, and she could hear him humming some pop song—was it "Unbreak My Heart"?—through the bubbly muffling of brushing his teeth. She had just finished putting away the groceries when the lights went out, and he stepped up behind her. "Sweet Katie," he said softly. "You have made me a proud man today. Thank you."

Katie waited until he was sound asleep before she slid out of bed and tiptoed to the closet, where she had stashed the dozen bagels she'd bought. They were on sale, she had told herself, and she would freeze them for Ahmed when they got home. The closet was the farthest away she could get from—*God, help me*, she started to cry—her husband. The first bite of what happened to be an everything bagel—salt, garlic, onion—was better than having that king-sized bed to herself. The second bite, which she tore off before swallowing the first, was better than being as deeply asleep as he was. She tore and chewed and swallowed whole gobs of the dozen bagels in fifteen minutes, the violence a match for the violence of her mother hanging up on her in the phone booth on Paradise Avenue, Ahmed's murmurs that she didn't understand as they made love, the pretty little ring Ingrid had bought for herself, and her own bare left ring finger as she held a cinnamon raisin bagel to her mouth and ate so brutally that the stiff dough made the corners of her mouth bleed.

"I don't know how to say no," Katie told me once. "Things have to blow up for me figure things out." Throughout her life, it has been her body that she blew up so that she would have the tedious bumping back down the scale to reflect on her mistakes. She was working on how to say no in DBT and therapy that June. Her fear of loss was larger than her fear of whether she was the right person for someone else's purposes. As she described her discomfort in the humid heat of San Bruno's summer fogs, it occurred to me that she had yet to learn to fear whether that someone would be right for hers.

FOUR

July

Walkabouts, Totems, and Dream Fasts

It was July when Mimi told me the story of her YMCA Hi-Y group's D.C. trip.

The January winds of Philadelphia are not kind, but for once, Mimi didn't care. Her plaid skirt whipped under her camel-hair coat as she almost danced to the station wagon and her waiting mother. Her Hi-Y leader, Mrs. Kraus, had announced that the group was going to Washington, D.C., for the Cherry Blossom Festival. The Y had chartered a bus, and the leaders had made arrangements to stay at a Y that was blocks from the White House. Then Mrs. Kraus passed out mimeographs of what there was to do and see besides the trees along the Tidal Basin. All the monuments were on the list and all the museums, as were tours they could arrange and even concerts at the National Cathedral. The kids got to decide what to see in the thirty-six hours they'd have in the city. There hadn't been a lot of time to discuss it after Mrs. Kraus handed out the permission forms and lists of rules and what to bring and what not, but Mimi already planned to advocate for the display of First Ladies' inauguration gowns.

"And the cherry trees will be beautiful," she said as her mother turned onto the West Chester Pike. Dirty slush flared from each car on the entrance ramp. "Remember those pictures in *Life*?"

When her mom didn't answer right away, Mimi looked up at her. "Remember?"

"Yes," she said slowly. With her little finger, she smoothed her pink lipstick at the corner of her mouth. Mimi had inherited her mother's fine skin and blonde hair and she ardently wished for the day when she would have her own grown-up gestures like that. She adored her mother. She was so elegant, even in her pink ski jacket and navy blue double knit pants. "You're really excited about this trip, aren't you?"

"The whole Hi-Y's going, and we get to pick what we want to do. It's almost like going alone." She scrunched her eyes up so that the blue disappeared. "And when is the group going?"

The group? Mimi could read her mother like a map. She pulled her seat belt away from her stomach to take a deep breath. "April eighth, ninth, and tenth." She was too scared to say "we're going."

"That's three months away," her mother said, and lapsed into silence. "A Taste of Honey" was playing on the radio, and Mimi tried to concentrate on the music as she stared straight ahead.

When the song ended and the announcer started reading head-lines, her mother reached out and snapped off the radio. "Don't you think it would be a good idea to *earn* this trip?" Mimi's mom asked. Mimi looked at her, considering. She did a lot of chores at home and then some. Last Saturday she'd dusted the baseboards, for instance, simply because she knew Mom would like it. What could she do to earn the seventy-five dollars for the trip?

As if reading her mind, her mother went on, "You could lose ten pounds. Ten pounds in three months is very doable."

It was Mimi's turn to say nothing.

"That would get you within thirty pounds of what Dr. Keske said you should weigh. You'd almost be thin by the time you start eighth grade. Wouldn't that be nice?" Her mom smiled at her without taking her eyes from the road.

"Sure," Mimi said. "It'd be great."

Her mother cleared a shelf in the cupboard for Mimi. Rye Krisp. Sugarless cookies that tasted like sawdust. Cans of tuna. Her own bottle of Sweeta. Metracal in chocolate, vanilla, and strawberry. She stocked the refrigerator with skim milk and 1 percent cottage cheese, and Mimi got her own "special" dinner each night, skinnless chicken breasts or broiled halibut with a lemon wedge, salad with another lemon wedge instead of dressing, a quarter cup of rice, which her mother leveled off with a knife. When Mimi reached for a banana to slice onto her Special K, Mom informed her that a small apple had almost fifteen fewer calories and was a lot more filling. Mimi ate the apple, and when she was starving as she diagrammed sentences at ten thirty, she told herself she'd have been just as hungry if she'd had the banana.

But she groaned when she opened her lunch box and found a container of tuna and pickle, no mayo, three Rye Krisps, and another apple. There would be an apple for a snack after school and an apple for dessert while her father and brother had ice cream. She thought of the talking tree in *The Wizard of Oz,* hurling apples in rage at being picked at.

Mimi wasn't angry, though. Not really. She wanted the diet to work. She had her heart set on a bright red miniskirt and go-go boots for the first day of eighth grade. Even ten pounds might mean the popular kids in Hi-Y would talk to her on the bus.

It was with high expectations and a stomach gurgling with hunger that she brought the bathroom scale downstairs on Saturday morning for her mother to see her progress.

"I don't understand," Mom said as the red line settled firmly on 140, right where it had been for months.

"Her system has to kick in," her father said, and chucked her under the chin. "Mimi's a good girl. I know she's trying hard."

Mimi was trying hard. She skipped her afternoon apple, and she asked her mother to pack Metracal for lunch. Chalky and warm, it was vile and she was embarrassed to drink it while everyone else was trading bologna for peanut butter sandwiches, but Mimi was sure that on Tuesday, her next inspected weigh-in, she would have lost many pounds. Already her waistbands felt looser and her knees seemed more defined. How cool would it be if she lost more than ten pounds by April?

The scale boinged and quieted with the red line firmly on 140.

Her mother sighed but said nothing. Mimi stepped off the scale, her throat too tight to speak, picked up the wretched thing, and lugged it back to the upstairs bathroom. She went straight to bed and dreamed of Hydrox cookies and Nestlé's chocolate milk; she woke singing "There'll be change in the weather, there'll be a change in me" until she realized it was the Metracal jingle and switched to, of all things, "Goober Peas." That's another thing she might do if—no, *when*—she got thin: write Dave Guard from the Kingston Trio a fan letter.

But *when*? On Saturday, her mother knelt on the kitchen floor to better see the black lines that signified two pounds each. "It's definitely between lines," she said. "You've lost a pound, Margaret. You should be proud of yourself."

After two and a half weeks of starving in order to lose one pound, how could she feel proud?

Mimi stumbled on the last stair and dropped the scale with a thud on the hall carpet. The red marker shifted below the zero. Or had it? What if the scale was below zero when she got on it a few minutes ago for her mother's inspection?

The next morning, the red needle lined up with zero and, yes, she breathed a sigh of relief, she was definitely between 140 and 138 pounds.

Her weight didn't shift in the following week, by which time Mimi, hungry and tired of the bland fake food she was eating, indulged in two brownies at Hi-Y and had bought a couple of Milky Way candy bars to eat on the way home from school.

How could something that weighed two-point-five *ounces* injure her diet?

"You're really staying with it," her mom said when she refused the after-school tangerine.

The Washington, D.C., trip was in eight weeks. She had nine pounds to lose.

"Maybe it's hormones," her mother said. "Are you having your period?"

Mimi's pale face turned scarlet. "No," she choked.

That night she heard her father say that they should let her go on the trip as a reward for dieting, but her mother was adamant. "I'll let her go if she loses seven," she conceded, "but I don't want to tell her that. She's forty pounds overweight, John. She can't go to high school *fat*. It's a matter of sticking with it. That's what I've done all these years—"

Here, Mimi mouthed the words with her mother. "I'm the same weight as I was on my wedding day."

A few weeks before the trip, as Mrs. Kraus was getting ready to call her parents about the missing permission form, Mimi had lost three pounds. When she came home from school on Friday with an A+ on her essay about the caste system in India, her mother said, "I wish you did as well on your diet as you do in school. You know what hard work is, Mimi. Why don't you apply yourself to *this*?"

"I do!" Mimi shouted.

Her mother turned from the stove in surprise. She studied her daughter, her short, plump, blonde, blue-eyed girl who had such a pretty face.

Mimi studied her mother back. She knew Mom was shocked into silence because Mimi didn't shout. Mimi didn't complain. Mimi didn't whine. Mimi got good grades, sang in the school and church choirs, did her chores, and went along with plans. *Except for my weight*, she thought at her mother, like the lasers they used on *Star Trek*, *I'm perfect. Except for* one *thing*.

The scale, the scale, the scale! Mimi thought as she made her bed the next morning. If only it would surrender two more pounds she was pretty sure Mom would sign the YMCA permission in the belief that Mimi would lose another couple of pounds. The last snow was melting, she'd be able to go for bike rides soon. Exercise would help. *Please, dearest Lord*, she prayed, pressing her elbows into the baby blue gingham bedspread. *Just two pounds.*

As quick as quick, a thought came to her, surely divinely sent. All she had to do was bump the scale. She could be on it and weighed without Mom being any wiser, and she could say she'd hadn't noticed if Mom found out.

"Five pounds!" Mom exclaimed. "Halfway there even though I doubt you'll make it in three weeks."

"How much more do you think I can lose before they go?" Mimi asked, careful to sound excited at the loss but without expecting a reward.

"You're such a smarty," her mother said, and swatted her lightly on the butt. "You do the math."

Mimi stared at the dial. "One and a half pounds. Or two. I'll be able to ride my bike really soon."

"When do the permissions have to be handed in?"

"This Tuesday," she said sadly.

"Well," her mom drawled, "considering that A+ in history and how well you do fractions *and* your idea to start riding your bicycle, I think my good girl should go to Washington, don't you?"

"Really?" Mimi exclaimed. "I can go? Oh, Mom, you'll see: I'll ride my bike for at least an hour a day, and my grades will be high and— and—" She sprang off the scale with a backwards skip, searching her mind for all the things she'd do to squeak onto that bus and make up the unlost pounds.

Which, as any fat girl who is older than thirteen would know, is the moment one's mother looks down and sees the red needle below zero.

"Margaret."

Mimi's stuttered to a halt. "Huh?"

"'Huh'? Is that what you have to say for yourself?"

She could feel the color climbing up her neck. "What's the matter?"

"You set the scale back two pounds."

"What?"

"I see what you did. You set the scale back. Oh, Mimi, I'm so ashamed of you."

"I didn't set it back," she protested. "I'd never do something like that." She bit her lip. "Do you think it's because I dropped it?"

"I think you want to go to Washington very badly."

"I do"—she could be completely honest about that—"but—but—I didn't—I tried—I stuck—it slipped . . ."

"That you'd set the scale back is bad, but that you'd *lie* about it—oh, Mimi." Her mom looked genuinely sad, which is what made Mimi start crying.

"I dropped it, Mom. I didn't notice the number, honest. Reweigh me, or send me to my room without breakfast. Please, you have to believe me. I'm not a liar."

"I'm sorry, Mimi. I'm sorry you had to do this and I'm sorry that you can't admit what you did and I'm sorry you can't apologize for it. I expect more from you. This was such an ugly thing to do to me."

"I'm sorry, Mama, I am. I'm sorry I dropped it. I'm sorry I can't lose weight. I'm trying. I'll keep on trying—you'll see. I know I'm not a good weight loser, but I'm not a liar, Mom. I'm good, really I am."

My mother only ever made one diet bargain with me. I was about four years old, and she told me if I lost weight—I don't know if there was a number attached—she would buy me the *Mr. Ed* record I coveted. She didn't tell me how to lose weight, but somehow I associated apples with diet food. I remember standing on our clunky gray scale, eating an apple, and watching for the number to go down. It didn't, my mother gave up and bought me the record anyway, and I was bored with it in about a day.

I usually laugh when I tell this story, but I couldn't when Mimi told me she lost three pounds in the next three weeks but stopped going to Hi-Y meetings for the rest of the school year because everyone was doing projects related to the trip.

"It was searing," she added. "I was trying. I was a *kid*. I weighed about 140 pounds—I was heavy for junior high. But I wasn't ugly, not the way I thought I was. I can remember like it was yesterday getting on that scale. My word was no good after what I did to the scale."

Mimi's story is a bastard child of what I have come to call "original myths": stories we told ourselves or that were, in tragic circumstances, told to us, about our selves when we were too young to counter the myths with soothing Stuart Smalleyisms—"I deserve good things. I am entitled to my share of happiness." Original myths are not the cause of why we overeat, but they are the primal emotional reasons for overeating, the triggers attached to biological circuitry.

The shortest kid in her classes, weighing nearly one and a half times more than her ideal weight is Mimi's myth of a Good but Fat, Ugly Girl, and she's been struggling to get out from under the myth since it settled on her shoulders at the age of seven. It's a heavy burden to live with because even though she was fat, she also got straight A's; while she was made fun of and later left out of the prom-cheerleader-boyfriend loop, she went to one of the best universities in the country; while she is a physical disappointment to her mother, she has been a consistently thoughtful, loving daughter.

Each time we remember them, stories like the Fable of the Scale and other original myths jigger at the adult demeanor we have invented for the world, like a mosquito swarm on a warm summer night that starts with one bite, which leads to another until we scratch ourselves raw. Or eat.

What sobers me in Mimi's account is that so many of us were handed a supremely adult task when we were too young for insight or even sustained attention. By failing to lose and maintain weight, we failed adulthood before we learned the multiplication tables or how to use tampons.

Further, Mimi did manage to lose weight, but the rules of the challenge she'd been set had changed. It wasn't *enough* that she was terribly sorry or that she ultimately succeeded. Instead of teaching her a lesson about lying or about the patience required in dieting, nothing she could do to make up for an act of desperation was *enough*. By extension, *she* wasn't enough. At the same time, the torment of being forty pounds overweight, wanting to eat all the time, wanting to go on her youth group's trip so much, her wild tears and wild promises were *too much*. And so the original myth of the Good but Fat, Ugly Mimi took on additional significance in which one thirteen-year-old girl was profligate in appetites and short on values—or value.

I like to think of the original myth as a postmodern, Judeo-Christian version of the Native American dream quest gone wrong. It's as though the young Lakota boy, after sitting in his circle, fasting, and meditating for a couple of days, meets not the bear or crow that other kids encounter, but a not overly bright mosquito. Mimi, like so many of us, has met her spirit guide in one of those stinging, venomous, bloodsucking mites.

If the Lakota boy comes down from his hill a man, even with a silly protector, ready to tell his story to the medicine man who will both teach him how to use it in his life and add it to the spiritual treasury of the tribe, modern Occidentals spend their lives either getting over and beyond their original myths or living up to them. Often it's both. When she told me the story of the scale, Mimi was just back from a national conference of medical librarians, where she addressed three hundred people. She led the development team for access at Thomas Jefferson University in Philadelphia. But despite her telling her parents that she does not want them to talk about her weight with her, the first night she is with them on any given visit to their retirement community in South Carolina, her mother asks if she has considered Lap-Band.

Mothers and their daughters' weight is, of course, one of the primal stories of the last hundred years, just as domestic accomplishments and virginity were for a little girl growing up in nineteenth-century Anytown, U.S.A. The primary difference between these stories of pressure and nonconformity is that virginity is not work and sewing a pinafore is a learned skill. What a daughter whose weight is a problem has in common with that girl who might have stepped out of *The Music Man* is how much the fat daughter betrays her mother. "I'm the same weight as I was on my wedding day," Mimi's mother bragged, and forty years later she is still a size 10.

Likewise, Lindsay's mother, a Sicilian American who could well have turned potato-shaped after the birth of three daughters, used to say that her husband could divorce her if she ever weighed more than 135 pounds. Lindsay was a normal-sized child: it wasn't until her senior year in high school that she started to binge and gain weight. Her sister Janice, less than two years younger, was designated the criminal chubby one in the family because she weighed the same as Lindsay for much of her childhood. The pictures Lindsay has shown me make this label grossly unfair. Lindsay, slightly taller, has bird-thin arms while Janice's arms are as fleshy as most little girls'. The pressure was on Janice, but fat was so anathema in the family and so closely studied on the body of her sister, that Lindsay absorbed much of the fat and ugly myth.

The ugly part attached itself to her when she was four and holding her cousin's beagle puppy. Janice tried to pull it away from her by its head, and the dog turned and bit Lindsay on the lip. The three stitches left a scar that has made her self-conscious ever since.

The Longhettis are a close family, and a loving one, but Lindsay is adamant that there is nothing worse in the complex of parents, grandparents, aunts, uncles, and cousins than being fat. Nowhere in her stories is there a mention of what was considered "good." Pretty must have approached it: perhaps, like the proverbial horse and carriage, it belongs to "thin." Three stitches and the myth of ugly was off and running. If Lindsay's other qualities—her good grades, athletic talent, and uncannily intuitive grasp of computers at the age of eleven—were not enough to lift her four-year-old's fear of what would happen if Mom gained weight, her scarred face clumped her in a category that was also rejectable.

In July, Mimi, Lindsay, Wendy, and I created a closed Flickr album and posted childhood photos of ourselves in an act of archaeology. We were astonished with each other because the pictures didn't always mesh with our descriptions of our childhood self-images. One night we all sat down and looked at the gallery while we were on Instant Messenger. "What scar?" Wendy commented on IM as she looked at a photo of Lindsay lounging deep in a couch with a book. "I don't see a scar."

"I *know*," Lindsay replied. "I look at photographs now, and I can't even see it. But I spent *hours* studying it in the mirror when I was a kid, poring over every picture of me—when I got caught, that is. I *hated* having my picture taken."

Listening to these histories, I can't recall being tortured with what would not happen because I was fat. The things I liked and was good at—swimming, reading, playing the piano, living in my dream worlds that were informed by musical comedies and books—were tacitly regarded as the stuff out of which I would make my future. In my mother's defense, if going to work meant a loss of protection and security for me, it might also have been an example of how my life would depend on pursuing my passions.

It was also my mother, my father told me recently, who forbid him from harping on my weight.

Katie's original myth includes the story that was told to her of being six months old when her pediatrician advised her mother to switch her to low-fat milk because she was overweight. She was seven when her mother came home with a copy of *Help Your Child Lose Weight and Keep It Off.* When she couldn't help Katie herself, she took her to Weight Watchers. "It was so dull," Katie says. "I'd complain about it, but Mom would start in on 'You're never gonna get a job, you're never gonna get a boyfriend.' I mean, I was nine years old when she started in with this shit, you know? I think it set me up so that I never want to do anything."

A script like that can certainly dim a kid's dreams. Perhaps it's part of why Katie has drifted from job to job and climbed up and down the scale so much. She would like to go back to school and get a master's degree in counseling so that she could work with troubled teens, but she hasn't pursued it to the point of getting grants and enrolling. The "you're never" scenario makes such work pointless because, as long as Katie is so blatantly obese, she'll never get the grant, never be admitted, never do well in class, never connect with the people involved in her practicum, etc. She settles for reality television and eavesdropping on other people's lives.

The fat child, unlike a child who may be dyslexic or epileptic, or suffering from the latest learning disorder, often becomes the "problem child." The family wants, badly, to "do something about" her weight if only she would cooperate. And, because weight is a hyper-visible problem that reflects on the state or status of the whole family, other problems can be ignored or considered more solvable. This was Katie's case. Her younger brothers were in constant trouble for truancy, tricked out as punk rockers, carrying a mean attitude. They were sent off to live with their father while Katie went through a series of emotional traumas with her mother, who kicked her out of the house when she was eighteen in the hopes that, out in the real world, having to support herself, she would stop eating.

"That's awful," I retorted when she told me this.

"She had every right," Katie says defensively. "My mom and I are very co. I can't stand it when my therapist starts in on her. She was sick of me."

"Sick of what?" I asked, inwardly gawping at the sadistic thrill her mother must get from a codependency that involves kicking her daughter out of the house.

"Sick of my fat. Sick of my eating. 'You have to be on your own,' she'd yell. That was supposed to make me lose weight and fix everything. But I was eighteen, and I kept getting these roommates who were bad news. One kid's friends—he went to my high school— all tried to get in bed with me when they were drunk. So I moved back home and then out." She sighs. "I was always looking for a new kitchen."

I ask her point-blank what her original myth is, and while she doesn't answer the question with a story, she gives me the result of her mother's label of fat and too emotional. "I'm not good enough. I have such a deep level of shame. It's like a barnacle on a ship."

This relationship of mothers, daughters, and weight is totemic; the construction is from the maternal experience and ethos of the daughter's identity through the size of her body. Wendy and her mother shared a heart-shaped face and cheek-splitting smile that diminishes their slight lantern jaws, as well as a weight problem. In Wendy's cycle of original myths, fat "is all I can remember." Her voice turned hoarse as she talked about that time, and her accent thickens with the memory of other voices. "When Ah was six, Ah heard mah mother tell mah aunt that I was up to a size 6X in a tone that verged on horror." Unlike the rest of the AFGs, being fat was something Wendy had in common with her mother, who had also painted a layer of permanence or inevitability of obesity on herself. "My mom says she was overweight all her married life. But look at photos, and you can see she gradually gained through the years. She would say, 'I don't want you to end up like me.'"

How a mother "ends up," whether she's fat, psychotic, or a brain surgeon, is the benchmark against which a daughter measures herself. Wendy's mother, Ida Wicks, is not the woman Wendy aspired to be, explaining that the best way to understand her mother is to read

Eudora Welty's "Why I Live at the P.O." ("And if Stella-Rondo should come to me this minute, on bended knees, and *attempt* to explain the incidents of her life with Mr. Whitaker, I'd simply put my fingers in both my ears and refuse to listen" could have come from Ida's mouth about her sister and sisters-in-law at any given six-month interval.)[24]

It would be easy to say that Ida Wicks was touchy and hypercritical and lived to judge others, but that underestimated her approach to life. Her abilities to outline any and all possible downsides of any given situation approached high art. In planning to drive almost three hours from Williamsburg to her hometown of Hillsville for a funeral, Wendy was faced not only with snow, but her mother's quirks that are about keeping score and being open to censure. "I have to clean out my car," Wendy complained. "Mama would not be happy if anyone saw what the inside of my car looks like. It's so stupid—I mean, who goes around and looks inside of people's cars at a funeral?" She thought a moment and answered her own question. "My mother."

Wendy's childhood weight problem was handled with as many techniques as a Cirque du Soleil juggler uses to handle his plates. As the only child and the beloved daughter/object Ida could control, Wendy was forced to diet as a companionable joint project. Wendy has fond memories of sitting on the couch with Ida, watching *Days of Our Lives* while they dipped into a box of Ayds candy. But by the age of fifteen, when she weighed around two hundred pounds, her mother's dire spin on facts came to rest on Wendy's weight. "My mom told Dr. Waterman that I was the laziest teenager she knew, and he prescribed [the stimulant] Eskatrol. It had to be the worst medicine I ever had in my life. I was mean, vicious, and nasty, and I threw away the pills. It turned out Jeffrey MacDonald was taking Eskatrol the week before he murdered his family, which is information I always find cheerful.

---

24 Eudora Welty, *The Collected Stories of Eudora Welty* (New York: Harcourt Brace Jovanovich, 1980), 56.

I hated that she said I was the laziest teen. Now I say, 'Wow, I didn't know that there was a contest; I would have tried harder.'"

Along with the "horror" of her weight, Wendy had a severe hearing loss. Her teachers thought she was retarded when she started school. In the alchemy of fat and ugly, the next ingredients are lazy and stupid. Wendy had hit a home run by the time she was a freshman in high school.

And so the totems build, with the face of the daughter on the bottom, the face of her mother above. Where are the fathers in this delicate process?

As part of the over-135-pounds Longhetti family joke, Lindsay's father used to point at random women and joke to his three daughters and wife, "How would you like *that* woman for your new mom?" It doesn't take rocket science to see why Lindsay drove herself crazy with worry about whether she physically appealed to Jalen, or that, perhaps in rebellion against his physical ideals, she had been bouncing around within a forty-pound range for the twelve years of their married life?

Her father's own weight history was that of a skinny boy and young man who developed a potbelly as he got older. When his brother Ted developed diabetes in the mid-nineties, Dean didn't take it very seriously, despite being Ted's identical twin. Once in a while, he'd grill up a bunch of hamburger patties and lose weight quickly on a sort of Atkins diet. The pounds would come back, setting up a series of diets and failures that didn't inspire Lindsay, Janice, or their baby sister, Alison, with much confidence. Each Sunday, Lindsay and Jalen visited the Longhettis, along with Janice and her new husband, and Alison. Lindsay referred to her parents' house as "Carb City," not so much because her mother was pressing cookies on them as because Lindsay was always famished before dinner was ready and succumbed to the lure of dinner rolls or holiday candy to tide her over. She and Jalen rarely had that stuff in their own home.

While Dean Longhetti was a coconspirator with his wife, Wendy's stories about her mother would make one think she was the dominant force in the family. However, it was her father who ruled with an iron fist. Joe was a hard-drinking redneck who could lash out when spoken to, let alone spoken *back* to. What affected Wendy more than his angry drinking were his fears for his only child. Up to second grade, she wasn't allowed to go farther than two houses in either direction. When she wanted to learn to swim, he thundered that she might drown; when it was time to take the training wheels off her bicycle, he replaced it with a huge tricycle that Wendy rode only in the basement. What kid, whose peers are riding cruiser bikes with their banana seats covered in stickers, is going to race around the hilly Virginia countryside on a trike?

Ida went along with most of Joe's pronouncements although she won the argument against his belief that vegetables would choke little Wendy. She, too, was monumentally afraid for her daughter although she recognized, and was slightly jealous of, Wendy's academic intelligence. Ida was also, in many ways, Joe's creation. When Joe got work as a drywaller, the house was flush with treats, a post-Depression way of saying the family was doing financially well. At other times the Wickses spent weekends selling odds and ends at flea markets. A capitulation to clutter is another habit all three Wickses share. To make a narrow income go further, Ida took in ironing at a dollar an hour. She was a mastermind of the cuisine of the poor: pot pies which were five for a dollar, boxed macaroni and cheese, noodles over toast— and her famous gravy. Wendy's spending money as she got older came from the fair prizes she won (once for ten cakes) from 4-H.

Wendy's original myths of being ever fat and lazy were fleshed out by the shame of not doing what her friends did, of being tethered to home, of being taught fear, and by the isolation these strictures imposed. Add to that her hearing loss and the bookishness that separated her from her hillbilly family, and the young woman who went away to college in Farmville had abilities and ironies but little ambition. "I had decided to be a journalist and never considered anything else, but I lacked the desire and fire to do extracurricular things to make my career happen, and I graduated during the worst recession, 1981."

She met Leo Hostenburg when she moved to Williamsburg after college and took a secretarial job in the law school at William and Mary. The courtship was dull but steady, and he never mentioned her weight or winced at her shopping habits that rapidly built up her credit card debt. He was getting his master's degree in social work, and Wendy trusted that he would never belittle her or rage at her. How could she have foreseen the self-blame she would heap on herself over his benign neglect?

Hiding one's light under the bushel of fat can be harder labor than the shame and discomfort of obesity. Wendy is always apologizing. She takes people—friends, her parents, men—too personally, becoming unctuous and ingratiating. This behavior drives her friends and potential lovers to distraction—and sometimes away. There's an old joke about how many Jewish mothers it takes to change a lightbulb that ends in "Never mind. I'll just sit here in the dark, all by myself . . ." and Wendy, when she doesn't feel she's getting enough attention or approval, is known to display that feint. She stalks her ex-boyfriends on the Internet only to dissolve into her innate belief that no one can love her for herself. What Wendy's "self" is remains buried in a tangle of ideas she hasn't acted on or in the tangle of magazines, CDs, videos, and books on her coffee table that haven't quite coalesced into a talking point. The closest she's come to that inner place that makes contentment possible is her diet and her devotion to the gym.

Wendy's lapses of self-awareness are the mark of someone who was not fostered in an atmosphere of encouraged exploration. With so many rules, she didn't learn to believe in herself and was criticized or punished for apparently arbitrary reasons, such as being grounded when she was eighteen because she got sunburned at her senior class picnic. Wendy got the better of that one by displaying long strips of peeling skin until Ida's disgust overcame her anger.

But anger over exactly what?

While Wendy's father may have been overbearing and controlling, at least he was around. Katie's father was a compulsive gambler who left his wife and three kids when Katie was seven. Until he left, everything the family owned, needed, or did was at risk, putting Katie, the oldest child, on what she calls "catastrophe patrol." There was the time her younger brother had severe bronchitis and their father drove all three kids and their mother to the doctor. "Pick us up in a half hour," Sarah Monahan said. He never showed up. The four Monahans waited, Stephen coughing and in need of the antibiotics they would have headed off to get, until it was plain Mike Monahan had stopped off at the track and wouldn't be coming to get them anytime soon. Twenty-four years old, raising three kids mostly, and soon absolutely, on her own, Sarah Monahan carried Stephen while Katie and Michael hung off her other arm for the two-mile walk home.

When Stephen and Michael went into their punk-rocker phase and were shipped off to Los Angeles to live with their dad, Mike had hit it big at the track and was living in a posh house with a pretty young wife. Sarah remarried, to a man the kids loathed for his prissiness, and whom Katie doubts Sarah was in love with, either. The boys, who were in trouble with the law, got the better end of the deal while Katie, who was fat but reliable, ping-ponged between sharing apartments with strangers and the stifling coldness of her mother and stepfather.

Reminiscent of John le Carré's accounts of his conman father, Mike Monahan was a charmer, without a bad word for anyone. "He's the only one who didn't mention my weight," Katie says, "and he always mentioned that he didn't mention my weight. He didn't love me enough, and he didn't love me often enough. He was good with sound bites and so am I, but while everyone loved him, I am such a loser. My depression is too much for people."

Too much. Not enough. Four words that resonate throughout our days and on our blogs, tickling the urge to eat, to recede to the small dark place that resides between the determination to seek our destiny and the deprivation-induced dream that provides the road map for it. When an Australian aborigine reaches adolescence, he undertakes a walkabout, a journey that retraces his ancestors' most significant events. In looking at the dynamics of our parents and families, we, too, undertake such a quest. Sometimes we have to go back another generation to understand what happened in that place where we are first taught what love is.

Mimi's mother lost her own mother at age eleven, and Mimi wonders if part of her mother's exactitude came from not having been shown how to be a mother. When Wendy looks back another generation, she has to consider the effect of parents who come from two different Southern social strata of what she calls "good country folk." Her paternal grandparents were tenant farmers who moved around a lot and didn't have indoor plumbing until the end of their lives. Her father didn't have much of a parenting example to follow, and her mother, one or two social steps up from her husband, has a sense of superiority in small things (her yard versus the yard across the street, a bargain she found that a friend didn't) that contributes to her meanness and judgments. Wendy reflects on the thin ice of tempers that she grew up among, and I know the next thing she'll say, in a voice that was bested long ago, is, "But what can you do?"

Of course our families push our buttons. They're the ones who installed them. Those first reasons for overeating, seen in a context of rebellion against, or adjustment to, our families, provide names for the buttons or triggers. We spend much of our adulthood trying to understand the reasons, triggers, and buttons of our compulsions. We turn to therapy, twelve-step programs, journaling, gyms, yoga, meditation, New Age gurus, church, Wicca, and the world of blogs, safe places for the ancient pain of our original myths and the selves we have made from them.

In the end, though, we eat. Food is companionship and a stand-in for love. We overeat to fill the not-enoughs. Thus, in part, fat becomes a rebellion against what is expected us of us, and a wall of excuses. The chemicals of sugar and fat subdue pains and fears.

As Lia, my Freudian Amazon reader wrote one day, "My inner fat woman is someone who uses my body to communicate with the world. She uses my fat body to silently scream: 'Help! Something's wrong with my life! I don't know what it is, but I am unhappy!' She is frequently the beacon of my discontent, arriving there years before my feeble mind can catch up. I wish she would learn to use her voice instead of my body to express herself. I honor my inner fat woman for the attempts she has made to manage emotional pain she knew no other way to assuage and for her attempts to have someone pay attention to her real experience.

"She is not my enemy. She is my clue."

Do our histories *make* us fat?

No. Our histories only provide some of the reasons to eat. Our fat is the billboard of those reasons, and our relapses are statements of the irresolution of those reasons. The great question, then, is what comes first, settling the score between the rivals of love and hate that rage in our hearts or, somehow, muffling the pulsing, yawning *want* of the next bite, the next hit that will take us to that fetal overfull place in which we are alive without living. Is our primary responsibility to our pasts or to the abstention and discipline in the moment? In the Angry Fat Girls' year of eating dangerously, everything we put in our mouths was an answer to those questions, even when we wanted, badly, to live up to the moment.

FIVE

August
Writing the Body

Mimi had a revelation, she wrote me in IM that August. "It's my decision whether to be happy or unhappy," she announced. The day before, her boss had asked her if she was happy. She was taken aback by the question, partly because he didn't frame it in reference to her job. "I don't usually think of myself as happy or unhappy, mostly busy or tired or fat or whatever—but not happy. If I can look beyond the cookie I shouldn't eat or what I didn't get done at the office, maybe I can start to get a life."

When did the phrase "get a life" come into currency? It's a concept I struggle with, too. I want my days to be as thick as the air the day Mimi and I bumped into each other online, a hot afternoon before storms rolled in. I envision days of joyful writing, a bed of basil and tomatoes to tend, time to read the *Times* and listen to NPR, going swimming and lifting weights at the gym, studying guidebooks for a trip to Prague, taking my dog down to the pond an hour before sunset, and discussing Almodóvar with close friends in the evening as the candles sputter in their own wax.

"We," I IM'd back, meaning the Angry Fat Girls, "all need a life." I thought a moment and added, "Except Lindsay. Lindsay has a life."

"Lindsay is whole," Mimi wrote back.

Whole, I mused as I headed out to the kitchen to make the salad that would be my second abstinent meal of the day. Intact. Entire. Boundaried. Separate but holding the possibility of being part of. Distinct parts tossed together to make a new thing.

Mimi and I were right. Lindsay is whole, and she has a life.

Lindsay worked hard to claim and expand her life and herself. I knew that because, starting in late July, I was part of it each morning in an eight thirty phone call she made while walking to campus. We had decided to commit each day's writing the way I committed my food to my sponsor. It gave us a chance to talk about the knots we'd encountered in our work, what we planned to do after we put in our time at the computer, what we were reading, and what the other AFGs were up to. I heard about her campus job in information technology and friends from women's studies, the yoga class she was taking, and what her plans were for the weekend.

I always had a lot to say about my writing and the dogs and the girls, but it wasn't a very broad spectrum of subjects.

Spectrum, I decided, is part of wholeness.

The morning after my IM talk with Mimi, I stepped on the scale and it settled at 220 pounds. "Well," I said out loud. "At least I have twenty pounds of safety."

Wha—? I was surprised at my automatic reaction to the number. I had seventy pounds to go before I would fit into my thinnest clothes, a long way and a long time, but my safety would, at two hundred pounds, diminish exponentially at every decade.

Every dieter has some size or number that means slipping into Hazmat. I'd be on the other side of "very fat." When I got thinner, people would take me more seriously and so I would also have to take myself more seriously. Which was scarier?

In the slow simmer of the library, Mimi was able to bring her lunch and walk over to the biopond to eat amid the butterflies that thrived in the Joe Pye weed. She had lost eight pounds since the March Weight Watchers weigh-in, and she was feeling good about how baggy some of her tunics were and how much improved her spirits were. Her Angry Fat Girlz posts were about "having just one" or "just a taste," about eating consciously, the way she did in the Penn gardens. On her own blog, she often posted recipes handed out by her Weight Watchers leader. That summer she was in love with what I called "puddurt," a mixture of thirty-two ounces of yogurt and a package of whatever flavor of sugar-free instant pudding she was in the mood for.

With a bum knee, Mimi was not able to exercise, but she was gunning to be the poster girl for Weight Watchers.

August in Virginia is beyond anything Philadelphia's notoriously vile weather can dream up. Wendy was taking the thick heat as a personal insult to add to the injuries of dating.

"Why is it that first dates never happen on weekend nights," she lamented to me as she drove home from work. Come Friday, she found herself at loose ends. Her best friend, Susan, a fellow secretary from the days Wendy worked at the library, was married, and it had come as something of a shock in the last two years when Wendy realized she really didn't have any other friends in town. She began going to the gym around seven p.m. on weekends. Like Mimi's library, the college gym was drowsier with the absence of a full student body. Ten minutes on the treadmill would show up as an "at least" clause in her blog when she recounted having twelve tortilla chips, four ounces of cheese, and a can of non-fat refried beans for supper. The next day, she would undereat and soon turn up with a loss and news of a pair of size 18 trousers.

"That's *not* Weight Watchers," Mimi said when we talked about Wendy's progress.

"I wonder which credit card had room for the pants?" I said to Lindsay as we drank coffee in our separate states.

Katie was drifting. Her weight loss was slow on her new plan—under thirty pounds in two months.[25] She was supposed to meet weekly with her sponsor to do step work, but she didn't like the way her sponsor's house smelled. Confusing matters more, she was reading a new diet book and becoming convinced that there was nothing wrong with a single piece of dark chocolate every day. I worried at the folly in this thinking but was glad to hear some good news from her: an ex-boss had called to ask if she would consider joining his franchising company, Pet Luv, and despite her freaking out about going to the interview at over four hundred pounds, he'd offered her a contract and she'd begun making sales within the week.

By August, Lindsay showed steady progress in a nifty bar graph on her personal blog, I Hate Carrot Sticks. At 168 pounds, she was shrinking out of her clothes while maintaining a continuum of activities. She showed up online at night less often because she was working on her dissertation about women in Texas politics. Her blog recounted weekly lunches with a friend and taking her father to the Spiritualist Church where she was learning to trust her hunches. In the spirit of wanting to share more of herself than her blog contributions, Lindsay posted photos on our Flickr site of her walk to campus, through woodsy fields and along streets of apartments. We got to see her yellow deep-porched two-story house surrounded by purple pansies and the sleepy willows along the Cuyahoga River where she walked with Jalen in the evening. Mimi, , Wendy, and I had mental pictures of her daily life and it inspired us to do the same thing.

The rest of us didn't have this steady stream of quiet activities moving through our weeks. Being married helped, as did living a half hour from her parents. But it was more than that. Lindsay was regular

---

25 It's important to keep in mind that standing up from a chair, at four hundred pounds, is the equivalent of five or ten squat-thrusts, which is exactly the motion involved. The heavier one is, the more weight one loses.

in her habits, and she enjoyed them—loved the gossip in the IT office where she worked, the accomplishment of sweat, her dad's corny jokes as they sat by the pool. It made me wonder, is she whole because she has a life, or does she have a life because she's whole?

And what does *whole* mean? I emailed Lindsay about Mimi's comments on her wholeness and asked what she thought about it. "It works, I guess," she wrote. "But my own issues—and working on them—is part of living authentically, too."

Her answer was a perfect Lindsayism: physical, intellectual, emotional, spiritual, political, and snark. I laughed out loud when I read it.

Of course Lindsay had read Simone de Beauvoir's *Pyrrhus and Cinéas*, she had studied the questions of the individual's right to be what she desires to be, how to live passionately, and how people can live in mutual freedom. She knew that in the realm beyond Dr. Phil ("... all of the things that are uniquely yours and need expression, rather than what you believe you are supposed to be and do")[26] authenticity is as political as it is personal. The "authentic life" comes from recognizing and acting on one's needs and heart fires while recognizing other's right do the same. Rather than pretzeling oneself to conform to social or family standards, one is a renegade. Lindsay worked hard at authenticity and had made great strides. The lady politicians of Texas who were her dissertation topic would approve entirely.

Of course, authentic does not mean unassailable. When authentic is stressed to its breaking point, you can fall back on having a life of routine. Or you can fall back on Long Island Iced Teas, the StairMaster, shopping, reality TV, therapy, antidepressants, or self-help bibles.

Or you can fall back on food.

Which is, for some of us, pretty much the end of living any kind of life at all. All five of us have spent vast amounts of time in that

---

26 "Defining Your Authentic Self," Dr. Phil, http://www.drphil.com/articles/article/73 (accessed).

place, helpless to break out. It is a lonely state, the fat woman and the food and her groaning, aching, widening body. Lindsay had been in that mute place of pain three times, between college graduation and graduate school, and twice when she found herself not so much a wife and lover as a mother, worrying about her husband's self-destructive behavior as though he were fifteen, and a diagnostician, frantically matching up symptoms to diseases. Expanding herself (her abilities, interests, ambitions, spirituality, friendships) as she defined the boundaries of self (where those moments of living most contentedly and in the most awareness bumped up against the bigger world of money, husband, academia, and family) was her ticket out of continuing to gain weight. Perhaps it's one of the great literary paradigms of the chubby heroine.

"I had continued to grow," Victoria Ransom, the narrator of Carol Dawson's *Body of Knowledge* says of being the last of a dynasty whittled away over the course of a three-generation vendetta.

> At first this puzzled me—where was the new material coming from? But then I realized that every book I read covering the familiar themes (*Paradise Lost*, austere Ahab and his murderous feud, my nightmare) added dimensions to my body of knowledge. And this last held the real fear . . . I was the only one left. The ultimate object of revenge. The Great White Whale.[27]

Victoria has been fed not only by her excellent cook, but also by the servants' gossip, of the family saga of couplings, births, killings, and maimings that had filled fifty years, while being stuffed by her scholar-grandfather with history, literature, and philosophy. As the last living Ransom, Victoria undertakes the assembly of the family history that her ancestors couldn't admit and confront. "They had left me here

---

27   Carol Dawson, *Body of Knowledge* (Chapel Hill: Algonquin Books, 1994), 404.

alone, abandoned, to serve as their monument." Her size—blamed on her malfunctioning hypothalamus and requiring the installation of a freight elevator to carry her from the ground to the second floor—is the human equivalent of a ducal family's coat of arms.

It is when Victoria learns that facts are not necessarily truth that her body unconsciously reinvents itself as she pines for unrealized connection in the gamuts of love, grief, intimacy, and desire that had not been included in her grandfather and nurse's stories.

> . . . I had lost them all, yet never learned to mull over loss, to mourn my vacant arms and lay my fingers on a face that had fled elsewhere. My appetite had vanished, I could not eat, living now upon air, upon understanding, upon the rolls and layers of the past's accretion.[28]

The ending of *Body of Knowledge* is inconclusive. Does Victoria emerge from her mausoleum into the world? Does she marry the man who unsettled her beliefs? Does she go on to write another book in keeping with her 180-degree-turn with food, called, perhaps, *Ghost of Ignorance*? We are told only that she is on the brink of venturing past the gate once the sun has set and that she needs new clothes.

I call miracle cures such as Victoria's weight loss the "Ordinary People Method": there will be an ah-ha! moment when some channel in the brain switches direction. Depression will turn to joy, cravings to satisfaction, chronic exhaustion to energy, aches to limberness.

This is what popular culture, which is where most of us live, sells us. In a culture led on a long leash held by the Me Generation, if we only understand *ourselves*, our lives will become painless masterpieces. Alas, in real life, the spontaneous remission that comes with understanding who/what to blame for our overeating and weight is

---

28 Ibid., 464.

dangerous because it promises that weight loss is synonymous with self-understanding, and it's backed up by shelves of books about emotional eating, intuitive eating, Freudian eating, and fat serenity.

Lindsay started to relax after Jalen laughed at her joke about Carp Lake. "Look, honey," she said, pointing at the exit sign off I-75. "I wonder what the honeymoon suite is like? It sounds perfect for us. We could argue over the one Diet Coke in the vending machine and the one pillow all night long!"

It had not been a pleasant drive. Jalen started out in the passenger seat, planning a run of the circumference of Mackinac Island after they checked into their hotel. His announcement made Lindsay step on the accelerator. They were on their way to Janice's wedding, Lindsay's "twin" in the Longhetti family lore, and the rehearsal was at six thirty. It was a five-hour drive with Toledo and Detroit traffic yet to endure. Jalen gasped at the car's surge; she sighed dramatically and from then on they bickered about everything.

She suggested changing drivers in Bridgeport but he insisted on Monroe. He wanted to picnic along Saginaw Bay but she nixed it. "We'll be lucky to get to the island by two," she said. "And an eight-mile run is going to do me in."

"Did I say we'd run the island?" he snapped back. If he hadn't been conspicuously not looking at her, he'd have seen her gawping like a drawbridge. She zoomed the loop around Toledo. The sign for Temperance made her retreat into a long, brooding silence.

On the ferry, the rush of air whipping her ponytail and making her T-shirt flap made anything seem possible. By the time they stepped onto Main Street, with its smells of horses and chocolate and roses, she was ready to make that run and be rested and on time to the church. When they turned up the long drive to the hotel, she was plotting whether to make love before or after the run. Or both, she smiled over the green, green lawn and deep shade of the verandah.

Jalen plopped on the bed just as she hoped. "That was an exhausting drive," he sighed, and reached for the remote control. He'd found a golf tournament and was snoring before she got her dresses hung up.

In Wally Lamb's *She's Come Undone*, Dolores realizes that the foundation of her obesity was being raped and overindulged in compensation and that she has fused the perpetrator with her father. As she inches up the ladder of these original myths—and further down the scale— her therapist prods her in such a way that the truth of her emerging body allows the truth of her past to emerge: "'How much do you weigh now?' he'd ask. 'One-sixty? One sixty-five? The ladder can hold you. Go on.'" [29]

Weight and eating are once again the metaphors for missing truth: "'So what if you died? So what? I'm not keeping your fucking secrets anymore! I'm sick . . . He hurt me, Mommy! He kept hurting me and hurting me, Mommy, and I'm not eating any more of your—'" [30]

Find the truth and it shall set ye free.

If we keep Dolores's trick of imagining her food covered in mold in mind, along with a copy of *It's Not About Food* at our elbows, all we need is our own *eureka!* moment.

The problem is that for each ah-ha! moment, there are many more uh-oh's that strip the body/life-in-process of its achievements and momentum. And for the woman who has regained and is trying to re-lose weight, there are more and deeper questions, about the body as well as the psyche, than sudden discoveries:

· Am I meant to be fat? Is this as much a part of me as the color of my eyes? Is being fat being true to my essential, inner self?

---

29   Wally Lamb, *She's Come Undone* (New York: Washington Square Press, 1992), 280.

30   Ibid., 278.

- Am I *doomed* to be fat? Will I be in prison with the feelings my fat inspires forever?

- If I couldn't keep my weight off on X diet, will Y work? Is an altogether different mind-set about food/eating/my body the answer?

- Did I get too cocky when I lost weight? Should I have not dated/ traveled/changed jobs/moved across the country/had a baby?

- Did I lose weight for the wrong reasons?

- Do I really want to be fat and I haven't realized it?

- Are the triggers to eat too compelling to ignore? Do I really want to live with those original myths that are so painful but which I can blunt with food?

- What, for that matter, is fat? What is thin? Did I lose too much or not enough?

- Do I need to readjust my goals?

These are plotlines not only of a growing number of American women's lives, but of the big bucks of mass media. Call it Chubby Chick Lit—or Chubby Chick Trash or Chubby Chick Flicks. Pop culture has begun to wonder, and to judge, how the world of fat versus thin feels and operates, and it's come up with a couple of basic scenarios: Victoria Ransom's spontaneous remission, Jemima J's conscious weight loss, and Cannie Shapiro's fat acceptance.[31] Are these mirrors we look into when we search out literary companions, or is real life and real weight loss different from the fairy tales we ante up ten or fifteen bucks a pop for?

---

31 Jane Green, *Jemima J: A Novel about Ugly Ducklings and Swans* (New York: Broadway Books, 1999). Jennifer Weiner, *Good in Bed* (New York: Pocket Books, 2001).

* * *

"Please be friendly," Lindsay hissed after the photographer had finished with the families. "It's the last wedding for Mom and Dad and it's extra-special."

Jalen pursed his lips but grunted in agreement. As though the universe had decided to throw its supreme test Jalen's way, Lindsay's aunt Carol broke away from talking to the maid of honor.

"Jan is the perfect bride," she gushed at them. "Such a tiny waist! It's really set off by her gown." She reached up and pinched Lindsay's cheek, twinkling madly. "You've lost weight, haven't you, Linny?"

"Yeah, I—"

"Jalen must be proud," she rushed on. "Has he gotten you on an exercise regime?"

Lindsay jabbed him in the ribs, silently screeching that he defend her. "Who wouldn't be proud to be married to Lindsay," he ought to say. Or, "What weight?" in a bewildered tone. He could go so far as to say, "You could use an exercise regime yourself, Carol. No wedding cake for you!"

He smiled at her aunt and straightened his tie, striped like a stick of grape hard candy, and said, "Are Jilly and Terri here? I'm under strict orders to dance with the whole family today."

When the DJ played "Never Can Say Goodbye," Lindsay went back to the hotel room with Jalen. That August day, on the lawn of a Victorian hotel on Mackinac Island, he was the only man she wanted to dance with, and he was dancing with every woman at the reception except her.

Lindsay cracked. Everything she had been proud of being and doing slipped away. No longer was she a grown-up and elegant woman in her black gown and grandmother's pearls, all but dissertation in women's studies, a computer whiz for Kent State technical support, and 5K marathon survivor. She wasn't Lindsay Maria Longhetti or Mrs. Jalen Easton. Once splintered, she couldn't face Jalen with any one of these claims to give her confidence or the words to explain her grief.

That night she was a size 14.

The operative word in her identity was *a*, an indefinite article denoting, her dictionary could tell her, a single but unspecified *thing*. So what if her gown was a loose 14, a little baggy across her chest. The gleaming black deep V-neck and spaghetti straps, she saw in the powder room mirror as she repaired her mascara, emphasized the girth of her arms, the expanse of her back. What had been an achievement—*almost a 12!*—made her look matronly, bigger than the label. As always, facts evade truth, and the truth is not a solution.

Sitting with her father and drinking warm champagne, pistol-whipped from going from feeling thin and desirable to fat as a thundercloud, Lindsay was smack-dab in an old literary paradigm: Jane Eyre getting her first close look at (the statuesquely beautiful) Blanche Ingram; Scarlett O'Hara greeting (the modest, bookish) Melanie at Twelve Oaks; Bridget Jones, feeling like "an enormous pudding," discovering her boyfriend's (skinny, tan) new lover.[32]

Bridget Jones is not fat, but she's made millions of women more aware of the company we keep each time we step on the scale. That she curses her eighteen-inch thighs may be annoying to those of us thundering along the sidewalk, but the reader can substitute her own agonies of the scale and the two novels make sense.

In August, when Lindsay weighed 168 pounds on her way to her goal of 155, she was not far off Bridget's ambitions for her body. Bridget reaches a high of 138 pounds ("... *oh God, hell. Beelzebub and all his subpoltergeists*") in the Christmas season near the end of *Bridget Jones: The Edge of Reason*, and a low of 119 pounds ("After eighteen years ... I have finally achieved it. It is no trick of the scales but confirmed by jeans. I am thin.") for at least three days in *Diary*.[33]

---

32   Helen Fielding, *Bridget Jones's Diary* (New York: Penguin Books, 1996), 153.

33   Bridget actually weighs 119 pounds once more, in *Edge of Reason*, but she is gaining weight from her all-time low of 114 pounds after incarceration in a Thailand prison: "(this must stop or jail sentence will have been wasted.)" Helen Fielding, *Bridget Jones: The Edge of Reason* (New York: Penguin Books, 1999), 262, 333.

Bridget's thirteen pounds versus Lindsay's nineteen pounds is not an unreasonable comparison, and the press was obsessed by the hows and whens of Renée Zellweger's twenty-pound gain (and subsequent loss) for the role.

But what, then, of Lindsay's high weight of 215 pounds, an eighty-pound gain over the years after her college graduation? Were those eighty pounds a metaphor?

Like Bridget, Lindsay was in her early thirties and had had career crises over what to do with her undergraduate English degree. Lindsay and Jalen were living together when she started a master's degree program in creative writing. She was a teaching assistant while he was making an unpredictable twenty dollars an hour at a gym and taking courses toward a BA in human movement studies. No matter how many times she explained their majors to her father, his consternation scared her.

"So let's say you write a really *great* poem," her father said, working out the problem like a logarithm. "How much could you sell it for? Have you ever thought about, you know, teaching high school English? The benefits are good, and you have your summers off: you should think about it, Linny."

Because she'd starved all day and binged all night at a high school where accessorizing meant a John Deere baseball cap, the idea of teaching made her hands sweat. Still, Lindsay had much of her father's pragmatism. Where was their future?

She quit the MFA program and went to work in real estate. There was always something to put in her mouth in the Century 21 office where every effort was made to welcome clients and build staff solidarity. The secretaries brought in homemade brownies and pancake-sized chocolate chip cookies, there were birthday cakes and seasonal specialties, and rousing choruses of "let's order pizza" at lunch, and drinking Petrifiers with coworkers a couple of nights a week.

She hated real estate.

She hated living in Akron, talking young single mothers into boxy apartments with views of parking lots. Her weight zoomed to 215 pounds and, a year after college graduation, she wore a size 16 dress for her wedding.

Underemployment is part of the Chick Lit formula, and it's one of the ingredients that separates Chick Lit from romance novels (along with, among other things, their generally comic writing, the genre's inclusive focus on friends and family relationships, and some sort of issue—i.e., alcohol and drug abuse in Marian Keyes's *Rachel's Holiday* or bad parenting in Emma McLaughlin and Nicola Kraus's *The Nanny Diaries*). Finding the perfect job isn't necessarily contingent on a major life change in Chick Lit at large, nor is it in life. Lindsay got into graduate school at over two hundred pounds, and Mimi has steadily worked her way up the academic library ladder during a weight career that has many hundreds of pounds lost and, mostly, gained. Still, one of the promises generated in fat fiction is self-fulfillment, the authentic life of following our bliss, through weight loss. Lindsay Faith Rech sums up this Emerald City aspect of Chubby Chick Lit in her novel, *Losing It*, in the journal that Diana starts writing during a break at the diner where (what else?) she works the night shift:

> ... she decided to make a list of everything she wanted to do with her new life. She called it Diana's "My Life is Far From Over" List, and it read:

> 1. Be skinny.
> 2. Find happier job.
> 3. Have sex again before I die.[34]

Diana has a counterpart in the overweight woman who is happily employed but whose contentment is undermined either by someone

---

34   Lindsay Faith Rech, *Losing It* (New York: Red Dress Ink, 2003), 70.

else's condemnation of her weight or her own misery regarding it. This paradigm can be snatched from the tabloid headlines and Hollywood reporters in any given week. Kirstie Alley, playing a fictionalized version of herself in *Fat Actress*, uses the casting couch twice to secure a lucrative holding deal from NBC but even so, she's told she'll have to lose weight before the network will create a show for her. From a "future so bright I had to wear shades," Margaret Cho was driven to physical collapse when her network informed her she had to lose significant weight ("They are concerned about the fullness of your face") in two weeks.

Cho's agent was appalled. ". . . if that is who they think you are, this show isn't going to work!"[35] Cho wasn't particularly overweight, and her agent's reaction was prescient. At the same time, it's a philosophy—*skinny isn't who you are*—that a lot of Chick Lit and Flicks, and tabloids sell their audiences.

Bucking that philosophy doesn't go unpunished. "You're going to go crazy again," Evie's fiancé warns when she sets herself to lose forty pounds so that she can walk down the aisle in a Vera Wang.[36] He's right, but it's not the diet that drives her around the bend this time, it's her success. Smugly delighted with her ultrathin body, she taps out her credit cards on new clothes and sleeps with her personal trainer. She's fired from work, her engagement is broken, and she eats her way back to plumpness within months—although, this being a sophisticated form of romance novel, the ending is a more mature, happily self-employed Evie.

Lindsay was immediately happier when she returned to Kent in the late nineties to finish her MFA and she liked working with the geeks in the university's technical support center. She lost weight slowly, and just before she turned thirty, she read Ingrid Molnar's *You*

---

35   Margaret Cho, *I'm the One That I Want* (New York: Ballantine Books, 2001), 107, 109.

36   Jackie Rose, *Slim Chance* (New York: Red Dress Ink, 2003), 49.

Don't Have to Be Thin to Win and decided that if she was going to plateau forever at 180 pounds, she could still be fit.

She set her sights on the Danskin Women's Triathlon. It was enough, she says, to try one last time to lose weight. "I wanted to get people off my back by being able to say I'd tried everything and nothing worked. I went to a nutritionist and got a food plan based on the American Diabetes Association diet. I started losing weight at about one pound a week." She felt good about her performance in the triathlon and her 155-pound body, but maintenance eluded her. In two years she regained twenty pounds, and trying to control her weight with exercise resulted in serious tendonitis.

She also cut back to part-time work because she'd decided to take her interest in politics and feminism back to school, this time for a PhD. Kent has a fine women's studies program, and Lindsay was consumed with excitement about her required courses, anticipating getting to work on dissertation politics, staying at the library until mid-evening, studying and talking with fellow graduate students.

"We never see each other anymore," Jalen complained two semesters into her degree. She was struck by how queasy his statement made her and how much an escape being on campus felt. She fell to thinking about how *heavy* it sometimes felt to be married. She had been the chief income producer for the first six years they were married, head cook and vacuum queen, the one who remembered his mom's birthday and when to use bleach in the wash. Each February she filed their taxes, knowing what credit card she'd pay off with the refund, and she did the bookkeeping as Jalen and Patra set up their personal trainer business.

Patra. Five feet nine inches of legs and suntan and long blonde hair, Jalen's best friend and running partner. There were times, of course, Lindsay'd been jealous, but they passed quickly. Patra had notoriously little patience for Jalen's moods.

As he preened in front of the mirror before and after his morning run, Lindsay thought she understood Jalen's concern for his looks.

It was one of his selling points. But while he looked great and was a talented athlete and teacher, he took little satisfaction in competing well or mastering a new form of exercise. Lindsay made up for it by being his cheerleader, clapping and yelling from the sidelines, a cup of Gatorade ready for him to grab, framing his instructor certifications, newspaper cuttings, and finish-line photos.

While working thirty hours a week and doing her doctorate coursework, she had jollied him through setting up his business, selling himself to new clients, researching the demographics of age and income with the probable form of exercise those clients would require. Home Fit held promise but in the twelve years she and Jalen had been together, whenever he took a day off, he collapsed into epic-length naps, acting nervous and cranky when he was awake. *It's only natural*, she sympathized. She, too, depended on exercise to keep her on an even keel. The difference was that when she'd had to quit running as she recovered from an injury or put yoga on hold when she got too busy, she still was able to show up for school and take care of Jalen, her family, work, and housekeeping. Jalen was so touchy about skipping a workout that she learned not to suggest alternate exercise or rest when he had blisters or a cold. It was easier to have gauze or chicken soup and Cold-EEZE waiting when he got home.

The next semester, Lindsay took a seminar in feminist theory and the body. A classmate presented a paper on exercise bulimia—overexercising in order to burn up excess calories. The profile didn't fit Jalen, who wasn't the food junkie that Lindsay has it in her to be, but it sent her back to the Internet, looking frantically for a word or a phrase for her husband's joyless beauty and strength.

In the summer of 2005, a year before Janice's wedding, Lindsay invited Jalen out to dinner at their favorite Chinese place. "There's this *thing*," she said slowly, willing her eyes off the lunar animal zodiac place mat to look him in the face. "It's not anybody's fault. It's not like . . . I don't know, herpes or malaria—" She smiled at him, prodding him to laugh. "It's more like alcoholism. You didn't go out and do something risky and then get sick because of it."

"Are you sick, Lins?" he asked.

"No. I mean, in a way, yeah, because I encourage it. I'm worried about you, actually."

"I'm fine," he said, his voice going flat, the way it always did when they talked about him beyond practical matters. "Those bruises are fading. Patra suggested that self-tanning stuff every other night to help cover them."

"That's kinda what I'm talking about, babe. Running on black ice, running after you've dinged yourself up on black ice, self-tanning lotion—"

"Spray," he corrected her.

"Whatever. Don't you ever think it's kind of nuts?" He looked blank. "I mean, do you ever feel like you couldn't stop if you wanted to? Do you notice how happy your clients are when they can squeeze out ten more reps or, like, the pictures you took when I finished the Danskin?" His expression hadn't changed. "Most people rest an injury," she plowed on, the air getting heavier with each sentence. "Most people are pleased when they improve their time or finish a race. Hell, I get excited when I lose one pound!"

"It's my job to be my fittest, Lindsay. It's a *job*."

"You know, when I go for a run or to yoga, I feel really good. I'm calmer, I can think better, I have more energy, I'm proud of myself. But you take no joy in working out. Your mood is always about how much faster you could have run or how much longer you should have stayed in the weight room. I remember how, when you'd get home, you'd still be hopping from foot to foot and laughing at people you'd seen or what you'd been thinking about. Now your workouts are never enough for you. Never good enough, never effective enough. You have a problem, babe. Jobs can be fun. You're allowed to feel good about yourself for doing it well, and you're allowed sick days and vacation. I don't think being fit is just your job, Jay. I think it's an addiction, and I think it's a problem you need to address."

How often the truth comes to us is in moments of opposition.

> "Fat . . . pig . . ." Rose gasped. "My God," she said, pointing at Jim. "You're a cheater, and you . . ." she pointed to Maggie, groping for the right word. "You're my sister," she finally said. "My *sister*. And the worst thing you can say about me is 'fat pig'?"
>
> She lifted the bag, twirled it, tied the top into a knot, and heaved it as hard as she could at the door. "Get out," she said. "I never want to see either one of you again."[37]

For Lindsay, as for the forty-pounds-overweight Rose, truth glimmered with the word *you*. In saying it, Lindsay took the first step in handing off the responsibility for how her husband felt and acted, just as Rose stopped supporting Maggie's waywardness. It required one step more for each woman to realize what she had done to someone they loved by holding on to that responsibility so tightly. Lindsay puts it this way: "My biggest battle is not to get control of my weight but to bring some sanity to those voices inside my head. Those voices can alternately sound like family members, like my husband, or just like a crazy version of myself. I tend to worry too much about what other people think of me and not enough of what I think of myself. This promotes a cycle of 'be good' and then 'rebel.'"

After their night at Bangkok Gardens, Lindsay headed straight for Melody Beattie's *Codependent No More*. Saying "you have a problem" to Jalen meant that she had one just as big.

I have to admit that I prefer entertainment to self-improvement. Chick Lit as a genre was a newborn when I was losing weight, and my journal informs me that I read *Bridget Jones's Diary* on the beach

---

37 Jennifer Weiner, *In Her Shoes* (New York: Washington Square Press, 2002), 168.

at Flathead the summer I went home to Montana and discovered I was a size 10. I looked to these novels for reassurance that I wasn't alone in being number-conscious, boy crazy, spendthrift, label-mad, and confounded by how to talk to my parents as I scrabbled to collect my new life. It made me feel like I was one of the rank and file, and it made me laugh enough that I continued to read it in relapse.

The woman who has vacillated between distinctly different-sized bodies is a multiple self-invention, sometimes hidden in a mansion of fat, sometimes naked in the truth of what she looks like, retaining her obesity long after she's thin by having to hide, minimize, or remove the damages weight and dieting have wrought on her body. The mental states of thin and fat are even slower to change.

Consider *Lady Oracle*, one of the first serious attempts to consider how weight loss turns a woman into a double agent:

> Suddenly I was down to the required weight, and I was face to face with the rest of my life. I was now a different person, and it was like being born fully-grown at the age of nineteen. I was the right shape, but I had the wrong past. I'd have to get rid of it entirely and construct a different one for myself, a more agreeable one.[38]

Joan Foster loses a hundred pounds at the age of eighteen and spends the rest of the novel keeping her childhood obesity a desperately held secret. Atwood does not tell us why her past is so shameful or perhaps we are meant to understand that Joan's weight, like Dolores's and Victoria's, is a metaphor of more family secrets encased (ah—"encased": one of the words of living fat!) in her tormented relationship with her mother.

Two of the bestselling Chick Lit novels that came immediately on the heels of *Bridget Jones* were Jane Green's *Jemima J.* and Jennifer

---

38   Margaret Atwood, *Lady Oracle* (New York: Fawcett Crest, 1976), 157.

Weiner's *Good in Bed*. Both novels feature overweight heroines but the characters, Jemima and Cannie, come to exactly opposite terms with their fat.

The first difficulty with looking to Chubby Chick Lit for the charms it offers the overweight reader is that it's usually difficult to pin down just what each heroine's statistics are. The novel may mention what the heroine weighs when she's fat or thin, but doesn't mention her height. We may be told what size she attains but not what label she wore when she started. Hints may be hidden in seasons as to the time it takes to lose a certain amount of weight, but we have to reread to ferret them out.

These are statistics that nearly every American woman calculates more readily than she does her Visa balance. When vital information is hidden or missing, it deprives us of the facts of what to expect from a diet and of where we fit in the pantheon of fatocity. It's possible that the authors of these novels want to be inclusive—that is, they want to appeal to women of all weights and all weight concerns. Or perhaps it's because the authors are both mystified and appalled by weights/sizes that seem fat to them personally. But because these stories stress weight loss, they leave every woman who has lost and regained asking, what does the world consider fat and thin, and what is fat and thin *for me*?

Jennifer Weiner maintains an active blog that crusades for her specific peeves and causes: the dignity of Chick Lit, writers who sell out, *The New York Times Book Review*'s paucity of new and/or female writers, etc. Author photos show a pretty, slightly apple-cheeked young woman. She has become known as the Voice of the Fat Heroine.

The opening premise of Weiner's first and most weight-oriented novel, *Good in Bed*, is the eponymous essay the heroine's ex-boyfriend has published about her in a popular women's magazine: "At five foot ten inches, with a linebacker's build and a weight that would have put her right at home on a pro football team's roster, C. couldn't make herself invisible."[39] Given that in 2006 the average pro football player's weight was 248 pounds, that would give Cannie a body mass index of 35.6, classing her, according to bariatricedge.com, as "severely obese."

Cannie's *attitude* toward her body, and how her life is affected by it, bears out these facts. "Twenty-eight years old, with thirty looming on the horizon. Drunk. Fat. Alone. Unloved. And, worst of all, a cliché. Ally McBeal and Bridget Jones put together, which was probably about how much I weighed . . ."[40]

The hitch in Weiner's setup comes on the following page. "I lurched toward [my bed], flung myself down, my arms and legs splayed out, like a size-sixteen starfish stapled to the comforter . . ."

Size 16 is the gown Lindsay wore for her own wedding and the black-and-white fashion photos she and a friend had taken as a lark. She is rueful when she looks at those pictures, but she's glowing as she and Jalen run down the aisle after their I-dos and her face is softened and eyes interestingly enigmatic in the pictures of her non-modeling portfolio. She weighed about 215 pounds at the time. She may have been deeply unhappy about her weight, but she was vibrantly alive with her family, new marriage, and girlfriends.

So a size 16 is *not* 248 pounds, especially on a large-boned, five-foot-ten-inch frame. A size 16 is less-than-ideal shopping in the misses' department. It's Ralph Lauren and Jones of New York and the scalloped laser-cut purple disco striped panties from Victoria's Secret that her ex-boyfriend lamented not being able to buy her for Valentine's Day—or the black teddy Jalen gave Lindsay, her size 16 wedding dress on the floor of their hotel room. A size 16 is overweight, a few months of dieting away from a size 12 and being able to suck up bargains at the end-of-season sales.

---

39 Jennifer Weiner, *Good in Bed* (New York: Pocket Books, 2001), 14.

40 Ibid., 19.

It doesn't take much imagination to figure out how these statistics make a woman who is five foot four inches and really does weigh 248 pounds feel. For the woman who has regained that weight, it's twice the rip-off. I didn't notice the first time I went down through size 16 because I was so focused on that and the next day's abstinence. Going up and past it was a mixture of shame and denial because I was failing— failing at maintenance but failing, too (and this is due in some small part to the low ceiling of most Chubby Chick Lit), to appreciate that getting bigger was not, ipso facto, freakish or humongous or the size 32 I wore only a few years earlier.

There are a number of these forty- or fifty-pound transformation stories, including Jackie Rose's *Slim Chance* and Lindsay Faith Rech's *Losing It*, whose heroines' self-hatred at what must be a size 18 body and rapid change of attitude as they lose weight makes for irritating reading to those who are truly hamstrung by their weight. As one woman posted on my Amazon blog after reading Judith Moore's *Fat Girl*, "What I found so nuts was [that she] still chooses to distance herself from the truly fat by saying she'd always been able to buckle her seat belt on a plane. My reaction? *Snort* AMATEUR. So what's her point? *'I'm Fat, but for God's sake I'm not as fat as those losers? I'm a 'fat girl,' but not the 'Fattest Girl?'"*

This is not to denigrate the torment of being more moderately overweight. Nor should the reader consider the canon of chubby chicks to be reality. The novels and the movies are, after all, more or less sophisticated romances, while the tabloids turn tales of caution and hope into scandals that often shake their fingers at the reader.

On the other hand, I, and other women who have dealt with serious weight gains and losses, find the mounting bibliography of fiction to be almost criminal in how it sets us up for the day we achieve goal weight or goal size.

I wanted, for instance, to throw *Jemima J.* out the window. I weighed about 155 pounds when I read it, 181 pounds less than I had three years earlier. I knew the loathing that Jemima, who weighed 217 pounds in the first chapter, felt for herself when her thighs spread into the adjoining bus seat, her wistfulness when she studied her pretty face in the mirror, how "'. . . fat . . . colors your whole life. Nobody wants to be seen with you, nobody notices you, or if they do it's because they think you're worthless.'"[41] Her shyness, isolation, secret ambitions, and crushes are the stuff I, too, had made a life out of.

What I know from the other side of fat is that a woman who has been overweight most of her life and then loses a considerable amount of weight will, even at the age of twenty-seven, have some sagging skin, cellulite, broken veins, and stretch marks. Her boobs will hang. To lose ninety-six pounds in something like five months on less than five hundred calories a day, she would lose her hair and smell of a butcher's shop, her breath ketonic from feasting on her own fat and muscle tissue. She will not know, her first time out in size 8 clothing, that men are ogling her. She will not have the skills, on that fateful size 8 day, to recognize and say to herself, "Bitches . . . they don't matter," when she overhears her roommates' insults. She would, a few weeks later, emphatically *not* respond to her second sexual encounter *in her life* with immediate unfettered exhibitionism:

> I don't want to do it with the lights off, or lying flat on my back so my stomach's almost flat, because now it is flat, and I don't have to feel self-conscious, or worry that he's not going to be able to do it because my size will turn him off . . .[42]

Jemima has some rough times as a consequence of her weight loss, but in the end we find her married to the man she has pined over for years, working in a magazine job she pined over for years, and ". . . no

---

41 Jane Green, *Jemima J: A Novel about Ugly Ducklings and Swans* (New York: Broadway Books, 2000), 263.

42 Ibid., 210.

longer skinny . . . Jemima Jones is now a voluptuous, feminine, curvy size 10 . . ."[43]

Excuse me?! Since when does a size 10 equate with voluptuous?

In its way, *Jemima J.* and other such "miracle loss" books are as dangerous as the memoirs of anorectics were to Marya Hornbacher in *Wasted*, who used them as how-to guides. They promise too much, too soon, too easily, and the stakes are too high. Lindsay would fume to hear that a size 10 is Jemima's concession to happiness. After much thought, Lindsay chose 155 pounds, a 10 to 12 clothing size for her, as her goal. She feels "skinny" at that weight—skinny and fit and energetic. *Jemima J.* is a slap in the face of women working hard to find the right weight to live comfortably.

The tabloid fat chicks are different from most of us because often they are unable to do their jobs as effectively or as lucratively when their weight balloons. Fame is also a curse. Lynn Redgrave, Lady Sarah Ferguson, Kirstie Alley, and Valerie Bertinelli have turned it to their pecuniary benefit by becoming spokeswomen for Jenny Craig and Weight Watchers, and Margaret Cho did a highly successful stand-up tour, film, and book about her experiences with ABC and *All American Girl*.

The tabloid chick who outs herself as honestly as Alley did has guts. One of the most hilariously honest scenes in all the chubby media I've looked at is the very first glimpse of Alley and her entourage in *Fat Actress*. Alley's hair and makeup assistant sits by the pool snipping out a Lane Bryant 1X label from a sweater and replaces it with another reading Prada Size 8.

That Lane Bryant 1X is truth. Every woman with a weight problem of more than fifty pounds *knows* what that label means. It is at 1X where Ralph Lauren becomes sheets, Jones of New York is found

---

43 Ibid., 373.

among the sunglasses on the accessories floor, and Victoria's Secret is a lip gloss in the Christmas stocking. For all the hype and irritation of Kirstie Alley, both as a character and on *Oprah* ("I don't want to have fat sex . . . I know what I look like, and I just can't see some guy's eyes going, 'Oh, my God!'"), scenes like the label replacement from *Fat Actress* speak of a humiliation that viewers can share (*"Oh, yeah: been there, done that"*), whereas the facts of obscuring pounds, inches, months, and labels make the process as esoteric as those epiphanies claqued over in *Body of Knowledge* or *Losing It*.

If Weiner's Cannie Shapiro (or Rose Feller with her collection of feet-binding Manolo Blahnik mules in *In Her Shoes*) is not quite what a lot of us consider fat, the five-foot-eight, 220-pound Kirstie Alley was. So is Dolores in *She's Come Undone*, whose descriptions of herself are plentiful and bleak: "My chin rested in a beard of fat. My eyes were small and piggy-looking."[44] Dolores is frustratingly vague on the actuality of her body, and it's only on page 398 that she finally states her high weight of 263 pounds. Until then we know only that she had dieted successfully to 138 pounds, a weight at which she can plan in advance how to be the victimizer and the victim, mowing through her therapist, the man she stalks and marries, the assorted friends she relates to through anger.

The heroines of Chubby Chick Lit are too often women one wouldn't want to know, larded with self-loathing and jealousy that may be lost with their excess pounds only to be replaced by smugness and revenge. "You're a beautiful person," Dolores's therapist tells her at the beginning of her treatment with him. "'Yeah, right, I'm Miss Universe,' I snapped back. 'I won it in the swimsuit competition.'"[45] Dolores's unremitting bitterness, sometimes dumb sarcasm,

---

44 Wally Lamb, *She's Come Undone*, 178.

45 Ibid., 256.

mistreatment of people, meanness, and blame make her one of the least likable heroines in Chubby Chick Lit. Despite years of therapy, Dolores fails to recognize she has a role in the disaster that is her life: her constant meanness to her mother and grandmother, her lackluster attempts in school or to fit in by behaving more pleasantly, stalking her ex-roommate's ex-boyfriend and marrying him in a forest of lies and silence about her past. Her weight, as I've pointed out, is attributable to her mother, who unwittingly indulged her after her rape, and to her missing father.

While very few fictional treatments of being overweight explore the emotional reasons for their eating (*She's Come Undone* and *Lady Oracle* are the exceptions among the novels, and *Eating* and *Now, Voyager* stand out among movies), some of the heroines at least shoulder the blame *and* the shame for their weight.

> Because, tough as it is to admit to a total stranger, I, Jemima Jones, eat a lot. I catch the glances, the glares of disapproval on the occasions I eat out in public, and I try my damnedest to ignore them. Should someone, some "friend" trying to be caring and sharing, question me gently, I'll tell them I have a thyroid problem, or a gland problem, and occasionally I'll tack on the fact that I have a super-low metabolism as well. Just so there's no doubt, just so people don't think that the only reason I am the size I am is because of the amount I eat.[46]

Insatiable emotional gorging is vividly replayed when Eleanor Samuels, a food writer, learns that her surrogate father has a short time to live, and she dashes out of the hospital before she has set down the spice cake that is Benny's favorite.

---

46   Jane Green, *Jemima J.*, 2.

I am hungry, so hungry, and I yank the cake pan closer to me on the seat, toss off the aluminum foil, dig a chunk out with my fingers. I stuff it into my mouth and lick frosting and crumbs from my fingers. I've barely swallowed it when I am digging again . . . [I] dig harder at the cake, feel the icing jam under my fingernails. I pull a larger piece free. I don't look into the windows of the car surrounding me. I know they are staring at me—thinking, What a pig. How can she do that to herself? Does she have no self-respect?—but it doesn't matter what they think. I've nearly cleared the contents of the 13 inch X 9 inch pan when suddenly I choke on a glob of frosting, the sugar burning like acid in my esophagus.[47]

It's refreshing to read such admissions after so many stories that treat excess weight like acne: a condition that happens *to* you rather than a condition you perpetuate by eating, for reasons of your own.

Lindsay can tell you exactly how feminist theorists break down in deconstructing size and the female body. The anorectic and hysteric's bodies are studied as psychological paradigms, while the fat body is an issue of political action.

How very stupid this is, and what a grave loss for some dissertationless graduate student somewhere. The overweight woman is as much an artifact as the anorectic, self-created in order to control a multitude of societal suppositions and impositions, needs and barrenness, social expectations and social rebellions. In the end, it's the tabloid fat chick, rather than the fictional hefty heroine, who really has to decide whether her personal failings contribute to her weight. For the differing degrees of openness about the causes and reasons for their weight that women like Kirstie Alley, Sarah, Duchess of York, and Oprah Winfrey have shared, I am grateful. "If I hadn't committed the

---

47 Jennie Shortridge, *Eating Heaven* (New York: NAL, 2005), 75.

mischief at hand," writes the tabloids' Duchess of Pork of her bashing from the press:

> ... surely I had done something else they had missed, and prob-ably it was worse. I deserved the beating. I had it coming.
>   And I was guilty: of mental cruelty and abuse, of attempted murder. I was bent on my destruction.[48]

All of us who have regained, or are gaining, weight are at risk of destroying the lives we worked hard to make, whether that life is still separate in pieces or has come together as a whole. What we have, beside the chunky monkeys of craving and the drive to eat more, is the knowledge that our bodies bear witness to our truth. If once upon a time my body lost over a hundred pounds—or thirty or 250 pounds—it can do it again.

A relapse into weight gain can involve very small numbers and still be significant. Lindsay was driven to lose fifteen pounds for the 5K marathon, but in 2005, when Lindsay woke after midnight to find Jalen's side of the bed empty and the distinct clink of weights hitting concrete, she knew what no one else had known. He had relapsed.

Jalen was exhausted and consumed with hatred for his body, mak-ing him sexually anorexic; his lack of interest made Lindsay feel crum-mier and crummier about her body and more needy of lovemaking for reassurance. "It was like, 'I'm fat and that's a turnoff to him,'" she remembered, and she turned to toast and cereal and grilled cheese sandwiches and a regain of fifteen pounds, which everyone in her family had something to say about. Finally she insisted Jalen go into therapy.

---

48   Sarah Ferguson with Jeff Copland, *Sarah, the Duchess of York: My Story* (New York: Pocket Books, 1996), 140.

"My *mind* knows it's not about me," she told me in a long IM session one morning, "I'm working on my heart knowing it, too." In therapy, she told me, Jalen personified his addiction to exercise as "Roberto," a name fit for the romance novel cover model's body he coveted. "He deals with Roberto. I just deal with him. If I see Roberto, I let him know, although I try not to monitor. Just if it's really flagrantly bad behavior that needs to stop." Lindsay has one of the few marriages in which it is the man who asks, "Am I fat?"

"One day I told Jalen, 'Being in a relationship with an addict who doesn't want to recover . . .'"

"And he said, 'Pointless.'" We laughed. "He and Roberto went into therapy fifteen months ago and now I'm starting to get to the place where I can work on my own issues."

Lindsay described the scene after the wedding reception to me two days after it happened. "It felt like an ouch. When you have a night where you feel gorgeous but end up sitting on a hotel room floor crying your eyes out, it's a real ouch." That weekend was an assault on the most vulnerable aspect of the person she has assembled (and remixed when the recipe wasn't right) in the twelve years since leaving college. In the storm of her disappointment that night, it was impossible to repeat the first three steps of CoDA's[49] that usually help her keep a distance from Jalen's sometimes callous or moody behavior. "I definitely saw my life go out of control because of my powerlessness over him," she said, the frayed edges of that night catching on her laugh. "He got it that he'd fucked up, and we actually had a pretty nice morning walking around the town and up to Sugar Loaf."

Part of working on authenticity is getting secure enough that Lindsay could confront Roberto and Jalen with what they had done

---

49 Codependents Anonymous, a twelve-step program for people who "enable" addiction in those closest to them.

and then move past the occasional bump in Jalen and her own recoveries. She didn't demand a scene of him begging for forgiveness to match the intensity of her grief at being abandoned at the reception, and while she was obviously pained, it didn't stop her from being in the moment of a sunny day on Mackinac Island with the man she loved.

"I bought a box of fudge," she confessed. "It's part of the experience of the island, after all. Half of it's left. Almost half. We haven't eaten all of it. It really *is* good fudge."

I was not the grand inquisitor of what my friends had in their cupboards, and I knew Lindsay had a million better things to do than punish herself or Jalen with fudge. She had Pilates that afternoon, and tiger lilies to pick, a church supper, and Ann Richards's speeches to review. Lindsay had stared her marriage—and possibly a life-threatening problem—in the face and had gone on to clean up her side of the street regarding it. That meant smothering her guilt, self-doubt, and worry about the future in order to go forward. It meant that the woman who married her college boyfriend at the age of twenty-two had had to map out her life beyond him and make her discoveries actual. *That* is living authentically. Her body was a piece of that life and her PhD would be a piece of it.

As is, one slowly savored piece at a time, the famous fudge that is part of experiencing Mackinac Island.

SIX

September

Twelve Million Women, Fat and Thin

Wendy Wicks has had the terrible misfortune of experiencing, and losing, a miracle.

No one knew what to make of the insecure, begging-to-please child who could read at the third-grade level before starting grade school but who failed her math and spelling tests. Her second-grade teacher gently broke the news to her mother that little Deesie was retarded.

"That cain't be!" her mother exclaimed, and turned to Wendy, sitting next to her in front of her second-grade teacher's desk, looking alternately at her spelling book and rubbing the scuff marks on her saddle shoes with spit. "She's just lazy, that's all. She lives in her own world. Honey"—she jerked Wendy's hand away from her shoe—"I want you to swear, right here and now, that you'll start paying attention more."

Wendy looked up at her mother. "Come on now, honey. Tell Mrs. Kirkland and I that you'll pay attention in class from now on."

Wendy nodded. "I promise, Momma. I always do."

It was hard to get Wendy to open up. Her parents said you practically had to beat the simplest answers out of her—did you dust the living room, did you remember to bring your lunch to school, do you want hot dogs or macaroni and cheese for dinner? It's not like they were asking her why she liked the Laura Ingalls Wilder books so much that she kept on checking them out of the library or what she played with her Barbie dolls or if she had a crush on a boy in her class. Ida knew prying didn't work, and it would never occur to Joe that a seven-year-old girl's life could be any more complicated than obeying rules and doing well in school.

The doctors didn't know what to say, either. One went so far as to recommend—very stridently, and in front of the child—that they shave Deesie's head, put a couple of holes in her, scrape the inside of her skull, and analyze the findings. Ida stormed out of the office and a few months later they tried another doctor, who gave Wendy a thorough exam, including a hearing test. He, too, was baffled but said she was in good shape, although a little chunky, and they should watch her weight.

One night Ida announced a Beltone Man was coming to visit. Wendy thought that was a lovely name but probably more suitable for a woman. Even so, when he opened his big square case and started hooking things up, she shrank behind her mother and refused to look.

"Nothin' to be scared of, Deesie-May. Watch me: Momma will take the test first and you can see it don't hurt."

Wendy watched round-eyed and intent. When the Beltone Man fitted her with the earmuffs, she did exactly what her Momma had done, just the way she'd been taught to do her chores around the house.

"Her hearing is perfect," the Beltone Man announced, and gave Wendy a big Tootsie Roll. "You've both got perfect hearing."

After a couple of years of failing more math tests and being pronounced a chubby but fine specimen, a doctor referred the Wickses to an audiologist. Wendy was terrified when he said he would shut her in a soundproof booth, but then she thought about the game shows and prizes of boats and Ship 'n Shore clothes, and she stopped crying before she'd started.

It was raining when they left the office, hard enough that it pelted down the last of the fall foliage into a squishy carpet as Wendy and Ida scurried to the car. As soon as they turned onto the highway, Ida started crying. Wendy slid down in her seat and scratched at the ridge of the upholstery.

"What'd I do, Momma?"

"Nothing, honey, nothing. It's a good thing, what we found out. I just feel so bad about you—everything you've missed, everything everyone's thought about you in school. But we're gonna fix it, Deesie-May. Now we know what to do."

"What're we gonna do?"

"You need hearing aids. All these years, you haven't heard half what you should. Me and Daddy are gonna get you hearing aids."

This is as much as Wendy remembers about being diagnosed with her hearing impairment in fourth grade, this and how the drive home to Hillsville was so emotional that her mother stopped and picked up a present for her, a salt- and pepper-shaker set of George and Martha Washington to go with her doll collection.

That gift is still a marvel to Wendy. "I mean, we were poor. I'm sure that one thing that was troubling her was the cost of the hearing aids, which they had to cover."

Wendy *does* remember getting glasses two years later. "I had no idea what it was to see things *clearly*." But unlike glasses, which made the world sharper, Wendy had to learn to hear. It took practice. Background noise was overwhelming and distracting; the cheeping of sparrows was equally compelling as her teacher at the blackboard; finding the tune of a Sunday hymn was difficult when for so long she had only the words. The audiologist suggested she listen to classical music to learn the nuances of sound and silence.

The hearing aids lasted until she was twenty-eight and died while Wendy was in a movie theater watching. Although she is a notorious spendthrift, Wendy still has not replaced her miracle.

In September 2006, Wendy was taking stock of the turns her life had taken, starting with her hearing impairment. "I compensate, nod my head. I have a stock set of phrases that imply that I understand perfectly well what's going on without actually agreeing to anything—I loved the episode of *Seinfeld* where Jerry's with the quiet talker, and he mistakenly agrees to wear the puffy shirt. I've been Seinfeld. Again, more fakery."

Memories like these can send Wendy's spirits plummeting, and it didn't take much that September to bring on her regrets and moods. After four or five months, the Angry Fat Girls were getting used to her temperamentalness. If she goes into a funk about Cal or doing taxes with Leo because after almost two years they still weren't legally separated, she goes doggo on us, writing, "I hope everyone is doing really well. I just don't have anything to say right now. I'm alright but I have nothing to contribute."

It infuriates us when she does this. She continues to blog on her own site, which is how we know what's on her mind and calendar, but her withdrawals from our group blog and Instant Messenger felt manipulative. We knew we were supposed to rush in and ask what the problem was, how we could help, doesn't she know how smart, funny, pretty, and fabulous she is?

Sometimes we gave in and sometimes we didn't. Mimi would cave first, posting comments on Wendy's blog and leaving her IM on so that she could offer the sympathy or consolation Wendy craved. I'd be next, calling for information about her weight history or high school boyfriend and find we were talking about how she just didn't feel comfortable with the other AFGs, the same line with which she'd coaxed Mimi into a momentary confederacy that felt like the partnership she wanted so much. Lindsay flat-out refused to indulge her, and Katie wanted stories secondhand. It was definitely fodder for gossip among us.

September was one of those spells in which Wendy disappeared from us. We learned why from her blog.

One evening, after she sank doing the freestyle in swimming class, she considered whether she should give up trying to learn to swim. Just why was she putting herself through this terror every week? Oh yeah ... Because once upon a time she didn't want to be afraid of going out with Cal on his boat.

It was a Friday night, and she had no plans for the weekend. She could be abducted by aliens and no one would know. She sucked at swimming because anything she wanted to accomplish, she couldn't. She'd never, in a year with Cal, seen his boat.

There is something of Alice down the rabbit hole in Wendy, who worries that, separated but not divorced and not in a relationship, she will fall through the earth, that she will be silenced until she shrinks into nothingness. She looks to people and things to take charge of her self-esteem, constantly lecturing herself, like Alice, not to appear ignorant or impolite, to follow the rules, not to overreact (in the middle of overreacting):

"'You ought to be ashamed of yourself,' said Alice, 'a great girl like you,' (she might well say this), 'to go on crying in this way! Stop this moment, I tell you!' But she went on all the same, shedding gallons of tears, until there was a large pool all round her ...."[50] Or does Wendy remind me of Tinker Bell? Watching the blog responses that metaphorically punch her on the shoulder and say, "Don't you know how courageous you are to keep taking swimming lessons? You're so lucky to have Cal out of your life. You'll meet the right guy at the right time: don't worry" are akin to clapping our hands if we believe in fairies.

The Tinker Bell pleas are one of the great bonuses of the blog world—if you can absorb the support. But like everyone who's ever

50 Lewis Carroll, *Alice's Adventures in Wonderland* (New York: W.W. Norton & Company, 1971), 15.

set foot on the set of *Dr. Phil*, until Wendy gets it for herself that she is courageous and lucky and a prize, all the reassurance, and all the weight loss, will never be enough.

Having nearly drowned, she stopped at McDonald's for french fries and a Diet Coke that was flat, got home to a hot apartment and hot cats, who wouldn't leave her alone. The day turned cruel in less than an hour, and she cried for two more, then called me, trying too hard to turn it all into a stand-up routine. "The pool is a good place to cry," she sniffed. "You can keep your goggles on or take them off or, if you can breathe underwater, just stay down there and be sad."

It sounds very much like the lonely privilege of not being able to hear or of living fat—faking that you're no different from anyone else. Breaking out of those privileges takes ear- and ego-splitting practice.

Wendy had met a nice guy online in the second half of August. I was more practiced at dating than Lindsay or Mimi, so Wendy marked me out for talking about boys. Mark was fifty, so I wasn't surprised when, in a fit of the pot calling the kettle dented, she told me he had baggage. At least Mark was fully divorced, but he had two kids in grade school. He was on the road most of the week, supervising construction sites. His ex-wife had run up an enormous credit card tab, which he was struggling to pay off, and he lived an hour away in Richmond. But he gasped with laughter when Wendy put *Fawlty Towers* on the VHS after they had lunch on their first date, and as she walked him out to his car, he promised to bring *A Fish Called Wanda* the next time they got together. The sun, as he kissed her good-bye, was heavy in a western sky that was the color of molten lead from the humidity.

"You're wonderful," he purred in her ear.

God, Wendy thought. *I love it when a man talks in my ear.*

"So are you," she said. "When will you come back to see me? Could you come midweek?"

"I can't," he sighed. His breath in her hair was a bit of heaven in the still evening. "I'll be upstate Tuesday to Friday."

"Oh." She kissed him again, with pent-up intention. He matched her eagerness. "What about next weekend?"

"I'll try. I need to see my kids, and I've been thinking about getting a weekend job, but I'll try."

"Just say when. I'll be waiting."

He managed, the following Saturday, to make it to Williamsburg in time to watch about twenty minutes of the movie before he drifted toward asleep. She led him to her bedroom, and he sank into a deep, dreamless sleep before she'd brushed her teeth. She crept into bed next to him and tried to count how many words she knew that began with the letter Y. It wasn't yet ten thirty, and she was full of nervous energy at the same time that she figured it would be rude to leave him there, alone.

She woke up in the morning with his erection pressed against her right hip. Mark stirred, and she whispered that the sex they had when he woke up briefly at two a.m. was goo-oo-ood. And it was, although she kind of wished he hadn't fallen asleep afterward. And she wished he stuck around for brunch at her favorite diner. But she understood. Really. He needed to get back to Fredericksburg to do some paperwork and laundry and help his seventh grader with her algebra before leaving for Annandale at the crack of dawn on Tuesday.

"I wish I could help," she IM'd him that night. "You could bring your laundry here next weekend." Cryptically, he responded with a kissy emoticon.

In less than a month, Wendy emailed Mimi, Lindsay, and me that she wasn't mad at us or anything, but she had nothing to say when we started chatting on Instant Messenger. On her blog, she referred to him as the Invisible Man.

Having made her grand pronouncement, she broke down and called me. "I don't want a full-time boyfriend. I'm tired of men."

"Good," I said. "Mark sounds perfect for you, then. You can take some time for yourself but still enjoy him every once in a while."

"I shouldn't complain," she went on. "I have a few nibbles online, but I keep thinking when they say I'm attractive, 'Did you just get out of prison?'"

"So take down your profile and use the time to think about what *you* want."

"My food has been *feh*. Not really bingeing but not good, either. I want to get under 250 by New Year's. I bought these camel flannel trousers at Talbots. They almost fit . . ."

"What kind of man would you really like to date?" I cut in. "Have you ever spelled that out? What would you like to do for a living, if you could do anything you wanted?"

"I need to get back to the gym," she said as if this answered either question. "I don't start Terrified Swimmers for a couple of weeks yet." She laughed. "I told my teacher he should call this class 'Considerably Less Frightened but Still Haunted by Fears of Drowning' Class."

I didn't know if she was ignoring me, couldn't hear me, or couldn't listen to me, but it was, I told Katie, who knew my blog cohorts only slightly, a classic Wendy move. She called about one thing and then reversed the conversation into yet deeper Wendy waters. Even when she called because *I* was in crisis, she managed to turn it back to her sadnesses. I think it has a lot to do with being hard of hearing and the social subtleties she hasn't learned as a result. She talks about herself because she doesn't hear other people talking about themselves.

On the other hand, it was a perfectly logical conversation given that our connection is predicated on losing weight. Down the rabbit hole of weight loss, the voices speak such nonsense that there is nothing to do but keep talking out loud until you can hear your own contradictions. The truth lies somewhere in between.

The next day, determined to make up for her nighttime woe, Wendy headed over to Five Continents for a salad after work. She flirted with the Cheese Pimp but only had a smidgen of Esrom and another of Ardi Gansa, which was so sweetly salty that she knew she'd spend the weekend wanting it. To allay the craving, she dropped by

Target and got a cute fisherman's sweater on sale for twelve bucks and a box of hundred-calorie chocolate chip cookie snack packs.

The sweater presented a problem. She folded it in the Rubbermaid bin of clothes that almost fit and, in doing so, had to look at the bins of clothes that no longer fit, no longer fit but which she liked too much to give up, and the clothes that fit and needed to be put away. The other messes in her four-room apartment popped into unwelcome focus: the piles of magazines and CD jewel cases and catalogs on her coffee table, the dishes she hadn't washed and the groceries she hadn't put away, the clothes tossed over doors, laundry spilling on the bedroom floor, books by her bed, the tangle of jewelry in the bathroom and on her bureau, and the sand her cats had kicked out of the litter box during the week.

"You need to make a list," she told herself sternly. "Get one thing cleaned and you'll feel better."

She decided to attack the clothes that were too big the next night.

"Too big," that weekend, meant sizes 24–28. Some, she decided, needed to be thrown out. The hard part was deciding whether to send things to friends from her blog community, go to Goodwill, or sell what still had tags. A.J., a Weight Watcher blogger in Arkansas and an Angry Fat Girlz responder whom Wendy had become good friends with, might like the purple knit tunic, and she'd lost some weight so a 24 would probably fit. The 26 green blazer would be great for Mimi and—hey, she remembered—she'd seen some hilarious Anne Taintor stamps at Barnes & Noble. Mimi spends a fortune on her hair—she'd love the bitchy blonde ones. She'd zip out and get a few things to add to the packages.

Mimi hated the blazer. It made her look like Dopey dressed up for St. Patrick's Day, the sleeves too long and a size too big, let alone the color. The stamps were funny, and she thought of the men she had stupidly loved when she read the one about running into an ex and backing up to run over him again. The lilac lotion was yummy although she stuck by H_2O products. But why, she puzzled, the yellow dishcloth? What was *that* about?

As the evening progressed, Mimi found herself increasingly irritated by the blazer. Above all, Wendy was loyal. She commented on every entry on Mimi's personal blog, Dieting on the Dewey Decimal System, and faithfully checked her Flickr album online, so she knew Mimi was wearing a size 24 and she knew how short she was. When Mimi posted photos of the Phoenix conference, she lavished praise on how the pink or red tops she favored added to the luster of her fine skin. With so much information, why did Wendy assume the blazer would be in any way something Mimi would wear? Did she think Mimi was *that* fat?

Mimi called and cautiously thanked her. "Don't you love that jacket?" Wendy rushed in. "It's hard to find wool blazers in that size."

Mimi's hand clenched the phone as she took a deep silent breath. "It must have looked great on you," she said calmly. "Green is definitely your color."

"But that was ages ago," Wendy said. "I tried it on, and I looked like the Sorcerer's Apprentice."

Touché, Mimi thought.

"I'm going to Talbots this weekend," Wendy rattled on. "I went to Lane Bryant last night because I had some coupons, and the manager said I needed to be fit for a new bra. Madeline—you remember, we grew up together—told me when I posted those new pictures on Flickr that my bra was too big but I didn't believe her. So this manager gets out a tape measure and it turns out I'm a 40 DD. I said, 'No way,' and she pulled at my old bra and said, 'You've got four extra inches you don't need there.' So I try on the bra she recommends and *guess what? It fit!* I take my coupons and buy four bras for fifty dollars. I've noticed the bra makes my stomach look smaller and that I have a waist. When I left the dressing room, the manager said, 'You need a new blouse, too. That one's too big.'"

"You know what Clinton and Stacy always say," Mimi answered. "It's all in the foundation." They laughed together at that. They'd spent more than a few Friday nights on the phone while watching *What Not to Wear*.

"Yeah," Wendy sighed happily. "I told my mom and she said, '*Forty DD?* That's almost a normal person's size.' So I'm going to see what Talbots has. I might even fit some misses' blouses."

What could Mimi say? She had re-lost nine pounds of ten she'd put on last year. She felt cautiously hopeful but was a long way from misses' sizes. "Wow," she said. "Good luck."

"Almost a normal person's size" are five of the most dangerous words in the lexicon of weight loss. To Wendy, with a severe hearing impairment and coming from 330 pounds, being "a normal person" stands out in sharp relief against "almost" and "size." It's so tantalizing, in fact, that it ignores the questions of what a normal and abnormal person are.

If we consider normal and average as near synonyms, we can compile a highly inaccurate typical peer. The average American woman is slightly less than five feet four inches tall and, averaging the averages reported in different surveys, 149 pounds.[51] She wears a size 14 dress,[52] a 36C bra,[53] and an 8 wide shoe,[54] and her BMI is 26.3,[55] which is one point into the overweight category and slightly less than the average American man. The average American woman consumes about

51   April Holiday, "A 5'4 Average American Female," November 10, 2007, http://www.wonderquest.com/size-women-us.htm (accessed).

52   Anne Ream, "Incredible Shrinking Woman," *Chicago Tribune*, July 29, 2007.

53   Anne Casselman, "The Physics of Bras," *Discover*, November 2005.

54   MIL-STD-1472F, Department of Defense Design Criteria Standard: Human Engineering, May 2007.

55   Cynthia L. Ogden, PhD, et al., "Mean Body Weight, Height, and Body Mass Index, United States," Advance Data from Vital Health and Statistics (Centers for Disease Control) no. 347 (October 2004).

1,840 calories a day, of which an average of 20 percent comes from refined sugars. Fifty-six percent of American women are on a diet at any given time.[56]

But Wendy isn't average, any more than the rest of us Angry Fat Girls are. Even leaving off how much she weighs, she is five inches taller that this "average" American women. If Wendy woke up one random Tuesday morning fitting and fit into a size 14, her blog readers and AFG comrades would never hear the end of it, and Talbots would be forced to initiate a lawsuit against the redheaded woman who had moved a sleeping bag under its sales racks. To Wendy, a size 14 might as well be a size 4.

Can you see my rage when Jennifer Weiner's Cannie wails on about being fat at size 16? Part of my diffidence is my problem, not Weiner's. Fat is far more an attitude than it is a hard-and-fast category imposed by the National Institutes of Health or the American Obesity Association. Cannie *feels* fat in her size 16 lawyer suits, especially when she looks at her sister, Maggie. Wendy *feels* almost normal when she buys a 40DD bra.

Wendy is the lone AFG who has not been thin as an adult. It's hard, to the fat outsider, to believe that the flood tide of self-help and spirituality books, tapes, DVDs, and seminars are selling to women who don't have a weight problem. The ever thin are trying to feel "normal," too, and who knows what haunts them as they leaf through Marianne Williamson or scan their nearby Bikram studio's offerings?

We who have lived on the Planet of Girls know that being thin and looking normal doesn't make us confident, loved, connected, or fulfilled. If anything, not having the present-tense scapegoat of obesity, the newly thin turn on themselves when things go wrong and with such ferocity that losing one's conscience to food has the rightness of

---

56   Psychology Today Staff, "Skin Deep," May 1, 1993, http://www.psychologytoday.com/articles/199305/skin-deep.

true north. Regaining our pulchritude is the reunion of the two last surviving classmates, you and your fat, who hated each other back in the day. It's—almost—worth the exponentially increased self-loathing, regret, and embarrassment, the reimposed physical barriers and life limitations, to have that familiar enemy to fill up the silences that the chorus of food, fat, and dieting once loudly drowned out.

On the other hand, Wendy has the longest romantic history of the Angry Fat Girls, including high school and college boyfriends, and a twenty-year marriage. She was at her adult low of 220 pounds when she married Leo and down thirty pounds from her highest weight of 330 pounds when she met and dated Cal.

Do Wendy's experiences belie my former belief, still held out of habit rather than my limited experiments, that a fat woman can't find love with a man unless she's willing to settle for a great deal less than what she hopes for or needs? Does a working definition of *fat* include remaining single or being part of a cartoon couple like Jack and the nameless Mrs. Spratt?

Yes and no. When Leo stopped wanting to have sex, she stayed with him for the safety and familiarity of a man she essentially liked and enjoyed. They had a dog and a house. She continues to call his mother every month or so. In our first conversation, a formal interview in June that was based on the questionnaire she had filled out for me, she said, "I used my extreme fatness to avoid situations. 'I'll stay fat and stay married and be unhappy and hope one day he will pay attention to me. I will stay fat and not bother to work out and be fit because "what's the use." You get old and you die,'" she says. It took years to trade a home, a best friend, and lack of sex for living on her secretarial salary and the hopes of 998 first dates.

Choice is the oxygen of the planet of weight loss, the very fuel that lends it momentum. What do we eat? When can we eat? How much do we eat? How can we justify it? How much will we lose if we don't eat it or eat at all? How long will we have to spend on the treadmill if we eat it? How will we feel about it in the morning? How long do we have before we weigh ourselves? What we "should" and "shouldn't" eat (and who says so is yet another choice) is many dieters' constant preoccupation.

These are the questions Wendy lives in. She blogs and talks about her food choices every other day. On days that she doesn't have to shrug off post-swimming french fries, she is sincerely and hilariously pissed off at the thin guy who had two sides of macaroni and cheese with his lunchtime meat loaf.

Sometimes the monomania of eating lifts. When we don't worry about what we are going to eat, that space in our brain is available to thoughts that can be difficult and as worrisome as the wanting to pop on over to the vending machines. Why are other people such *ass*holes? When is someone going to find out how incompetent, selfish, bitchy, stupid, and vain we are? Will we lose our jobs or friends or marriage when they do? Should we change jobs? Are we spending enough time with family? Mom's moved to a rest home—how will we cope when she's gone? How do we bear the loneliness and nakedness of not eating what, when, and as much as we want?

New questions lead to a new set of choices. Either we face the worries and deal with them, find new distractions, or get into a diet cycle of bad this week but a new diet next week will do the trick.

Wendy seesaws between the last two choices—taking a hard look at how she lives and having a week of slippery food—by shopping, justifying, and punishing herself. "I don't like it when I shove giant gumdrops in my mouth because I'm ticked off," she said of one sad weekend. Her options to eating leave her broke, with an apartment full of clothes, magazines, and CDs; obsessing over dating websites; and blogging about how long she spent on the treadmill and at what incline. Only once, in a crisis with her boss, have I heard her consider another campus secretarial position in which she'd be working with creative rather than administrative people. It seems as if Wendy willfully refuses to consider more ways to spend free time, how to express herself, or to find more fulfilling work. One advantage of having a lot of weight to lose is having the time to consider what kind of human being she'd like to become during and after the process. But Wendy is seduced by the numbers on the scale and labels, which are faulty markers of progress and time. "I'm not as fat as I used to be," she explained during one of her brief disappearances from the personal ads, "but I'm still not attractive enough for men in my age bracket. If I want to date a sixty-nine-year-old, I'm hot, but that's not my cup of tea."

Choice—in cute clothes, cute men, taking any flight because the middle seat is just fine, a beach vacation—is also the treasured goal of weight loss, whether it's fantasy of reality.

For Wendy, then, it's not so much that *fat* means being less lovable than it means perceived limitations, and her balls-to-the-wind attitude toward dating is, in many ways, a continuation of obesity, holding out the possibility of safety and comfortableness. She was, that August, twenty pounds lighter than she'd been with Cal: love is possible at any weight. But her driving need to find a boyfriend is the desire to get out of the mating arena where judgments are made rapidly and sometimes cruelly, to have someone to complain to about her job and her parents, to be rescued, hopefully, from her precarious finances, to be behind a male set of walls. Limits are what Wendy has lived with her entire life, from the father who thought riding a bike was too dangerous to working as a secretary in the same system for nearly twenty years. She could reason away Mark's unavailability that September by saying she didn't really want a full-time boyfriend, and she could palm off how acutely Cal had belittled her by hurling invectives about the woman she calls "the she-male" who bewitched him away from her, but their unavailability pinched an old nerve nonetheless.

Belittlement is one of the terrors that choice holds, and I think that's the real reason we don't hear Wendy talking about possible alternatives to being a secretary in the registrar's office. She had her bachelor's degree in journalism and would be eligible for her pension from the university soon. She said she wanted to write, and she had a million ideas for stories and novels, some of which she took to leaving on my answering machine, thinking I needed the material rather than trying it for herself. Her blog and Angry Fat Girlz were amazingly open and accepting places for her to speak out, but when I offered to help her with some of the awkwardness of her writing, she thanked me but never got around to asking for specifics. Writing is hard work and hard on the writer—she could expect nothing but criticism for years at a time. It's a calling that requires its practitioner to be both a perfectionist and a vagabond because the writer doesn't know where the day will take her or what the next project will be, and the failures inherent in jumping out of the airplane are her own.

That state of unpredictability and culpability was not for Wendy. For the woman who chooses to make her career an active part of her life, culpability and unpredictability are part of the equation of success. Just ask Mimi, who, as she advanced in her field and had fewer people to answer to, was the one who got blamed if something dire happened, or Lindsay, who would be on her own once she finished her doctorate.

Perhaps everyone, fat or thin, has the courage to face failure in only one or two areas of her life. I'm not sure I'm brave enough anymore to face the stress of dating or the decimation of breaking up. I tell myself I'll look for a boyfriend when I've lost more weight, knowing it's time I'm playing for, and with it, the hope that I'll be so secure with who I am that I'll be slick as Teflon by the time I get there. Whatever gunk men come with—kids, running a business, allergies, whatever—will slide right off me.

Or perhaps we don't pick our battles. Perhaps our battles pick us.

I was surprised how judgmental heavy women are of what constitutes fat, obese, thin, skinny, and freakish at either extreme. Ann, a nurse, based her distinctions clinically on rolls and muscle definition, adding, "Thin women have ease in their carriage and no stress as they move."

Gee, I thought, *tell that to my friend Kay, who broke her back but has remained a size 4 for twenty years after a long history of yo-yoing from a 4 to a 16 twice a year, or my niece Lisa, who so hates having to dress up that she looked frozen in her wedding finery.*

Lia, the Freudian blogger, responded to my question on my Amazon blog by writing, "Thin is sizes 6 and 8. Size 10 is regular (or normal, or average), size 12 is chubby, while that wearisome 14 is overweight. If you fit sizes to 16 or 18, you're fat, and 20 to 24 labels mean you're obese." A 26 to "no-size muumuu" is morbidly obese in Lia's categories, and after that you're in what I bluntly call freakishly fat and how-do-they-live-that-way fat. At that point, Lia says, clothing doesn't matter so much as bed linens and a Discovery Channel intervention.

These pairings make me think of how thin I felt and how good my legs looked in the sizes Lia defines as overweight. As I lost weight, I never, once, felt "chubby" in a size 12, and fitting a 6 or 8 meant, to me, that I could shop anywhere in SoHo or on Madison Avenue. I felt surprised—that I could be that small, that there is another category of clothing there—but not thinner as a 6 than I had at 12. Until, of course, I began *gaining* weight.

My friend B.J. recently came across a term neither of us had heard before for that bedridden woman who writes pleading letters to Richard Simmons: *super morbid obesity*. It's defined, I learned, by having a body mass of fifty or above. At our heaviest, I was one point into super morbid obesity and Wendy was one-tenth of a point into it. It's both a horrible and wonderful designation, admitting the blockbuster heroism that it takes to create and live in such hampered bodies and expectations.

Another friend, Monica, refers to brand names in considering classifications of clothing sizes. The obese woman can fit into size 3X's in department stores; the morbidly obese can sometimes fit into Lane Bryant's largest sizes; the freakishly fat, my phrasing which she rightly took umbrage to, can fit into some of Roaman's clothing and she needs help getting around. Like Lia, Monica thinks the how-does-she-live-that-way fat woman needs clothing made for her and is immobile.

B.J., Monica, Ann, Lia, and I were all obese as we discussed these differences. B.J. had recently gotten married. Monica runs a successful business that requires constant commuting by bus and plane. Ann teaches nursing and is raising two sons on her own. Lia has completed all but her dissertation in clinical psychology and worked at a big-city law firm while conducting a busy social life with her husband and a circle of intellectual friends.

How we live and what we believe, as if Wendy's contrariness hasn't illustrated, are two completely different things.

Despite all the caterwauling in the press and medical communities, and the screeds about fatties you can find online and in crude comics' shticks, being fat isn't what it used to be when there was only the Lane Bryant catalog and doctors who readily dispensed amphetamines and thyroid pills without testing. It's expensive to be fat but increasingly feasible, health- and fashion-conscious, and social.

It has been difficult, for instance, to ascertain correct readings from too-small blood pressure cuffs. Many fat patients now take their own examination gown and larger cuffs to the doctor's office, along with their personal seat belt extender to the airport. MRI machines and even operating tables have been enlarged and strengthened.

Fat travelers now have destinations of their own, tailored to their needs. Freedom Paradise opened its twelve-room Riviera Maya in Mexico in 2004. It features armless chairs and ladderless swimming pools, and staff tutored by psychologists to look their guests in the eye. BBW (Big Beautiful Woman) Travel offers size-friendly trips to the Caribbean, Mexico, Las Vegas, and Disney World, and packages catering to sports fans, skiers, and golfers. They also offer group, semi-escorted, and individual plans for trips to Europe, the major American cities, South America, and the Near East. The proprietress of BBW Travel, Jo-Ellen Hodgkins, is especially enamored of cruises.

Unlike other travel websites, BBW Travel features links to purchase hard-to-find plus-sized travel items such as fanny packs and plus-sized garment bags, explanations of travel clothes and extra-wide hangers. I recently received a catalog offering such products and more. I studied it in horrified fascination for the insights it offers into the needs of the super morbidly obese: raised toilet seats that will bear eight hundred pounds, convex replacement rods that extend a bathtub shower several feet outwards, roomy lawn chairs, and stronger, wider bicycle seats. I felt like a rookie as I filed the catalog in a folder, and I wondered if its patrons mind that the models, while more discernibly hefty than most so-called plus-sized models, are beautiful, tanned, sporty, and sexy size 20s with 48-inch waists. These models clearly don't need the scale that weighs up to a thousand pounds.

None of this is cheap, which makes fat good for the American economy by creating a burgeoning "fatonomics," as Daniel Gross describes it.[57] The increased premiums that the overweight and obese pay, often for no other reason than the number on the scale, are stuffing the pockets of major HMOs and insurance companies. Fat people are advised, both by the National Association to Advance Fat Americans (NAAFA) and the airlines, to consider buying either two economy or one first-class seat. That is double the ticket money for Delta for half the passengers.

Fat people may have contributed to the survival of e-commerce because the Internet is often the only way to avail ourselves of goods and services. If you want one of Yuliya Zeltser's delicious IGIGI evening gowns, most women are going to have to go online to make the selection. IGIGI is a smaller business that has been built on the understanding that fat women's bodies have shapes. The buyer has some guarantee that she won't shriek when she looks in the mirror and then scurry to locate something else and return the disaster for a refund. Such boutiques are featured on many blogs and online communities, decreasing the need for advertising.

Among the already-more-expensive plus sizes, there is another 5 to 10 percent price difference between sizes. The cute chocolate tweed sweater at Woman Within that sells for $34.99 in sizes medium (14/16W) through 1X (22/24W) is $39.99 in sizes 2X (26/28W) to 4X

---

57 Daneil Gross, "Economy of Scale: How Fat People Could Save American Business," July 21, 2005, http://www.moneybox.com.

(34/36W). A fat woman's purchases often inflate because of Desperate Shopper's Syndrome: if it fits, I'd better buy it because you never know when I'll find something else. Once a woman gets to those bigger sizes, DSS isn't frivolous. In looking at the OneStopPlus website that features clothing from three Redcats' brands that all fat women know well—Woman Within, Roaman's, and Jessica London—there were seven newly arrived items in 4X/36W. The washable suede skirt that could reasonably make the fifty-inch-waisted woman feel sexy is ten dollars more than its smaller sizes.

Plus-sized clothing is one of the biggest growth areas in the fashion industry, IGIGI's Yuliya Zeltser notes. Even the most coveted designers are claiming their slice of the pie—with inferior goods. Cruise the misses' racks and compare a skirt or pair of jeans with its twin on the plus-sized racks. You'll find a marked difference in material and workmanship. And yet I'm heartened to see that, up to about size 24, fat women can now shop many of the same brands as the thin. When I was growing up, there was little chance to make the kind of statement about who I was or wanted to be from the clothes I could buy. Now I can sate my fantasies at J. Jill (*très artistique*), Coldwater Creek (boardroom to ballroom in florid prose), and Eddie Bauer (another sunrise at tree line, ho-hum).

If only I liked the way I actually look in the toile skirt from JCPenney's or the quilted red silk jacket from Spiegel . . .

Among the sectors you might not think of profiting from fatonomics are the automobile and petroleum industries. In *Fat Chicks Rule!* Lara Frater devotes three pages to buying a car that is fat friendly, including the companies that do and don't offer seat belt extenders. These are products that Mimi, Wendy, Katie, and I have needed and use in common with the most militant Bod Squad Cheerleader. But the Angry Fat Girls pay more to keep fatonomics thriving by buying into some of the diet, scholarly, medical, and political industries. Wendy, Mimi, and Lindsay fork over a monthly $46.90 to Weight Watchers, and Katie and I toss a buck or two in a basket at meetings.

It costs about $1,400 a year to join the gym around the corner and just over $900 dollars to join the nearest Y (a five-dollar, subway ride away, adding $750 if I went three times a week), or $1,600 for a yearlong membership in the nearest Bikram Yoga studio.

I should move. Mimi's local Y in West Philadelphia is $567 a year and her closest yoga studio is $1,236 a year.[58]

On the other hand, if I don't get down to 180 pounds, which would put me in a size 12 and two points into the NIH category for over-weight, I'm doing all the thin, funny, well-read, tall, leggy, blue-eyed, self-exposed, talented people a huge favor: I am less likely to find a job or make as much money as that Thin Frances X. If I do find a job, I'm less likely to receive good work reviews and less likely to be promoted. If I have to move for my job, I will find it harder to rent an apartment.

The one-third of the American public that is not overweight or obese should be sending us flowers and Godiva chocolates in gratitude.

For the less than half of American women who are in normal bodies (whether they like their bodies or not), this is what it's really like to be fat.

Put on a pair of leggings or long underwear, and a pair of thick, knee-high socks. Pull on a T-shirt, followed by a turtleneck, and a stout wool sweater. Next you will need a pair of down-filled ski pants, a size too small. Last, add boots and a long, down-filled coat. It's seventy-two degrees inside but that's okay because you're about to go out and walk a couple of big rambunctious dogs in a strong windchill that will have you pushing against it with your shoulders as the dogs pull you in three separate, shifting directions.

When you stoop to pick up a dropped leash or a pile of shit, you will strain—against so many clothes and the trousers that bind at your

---

58   J. Eric Oliver, *Fat Politics: The Real Story Behind America's Obesity Epidemic* (New York: Oxford University Press, 2006), 60.

waist and thighs. You struggle to hitch two thick layers up in order to half squat to bend over, and you will grunt with the effort. Your coat may unsnap in these maneuvers, but you'll thank God your ass is hidden by it: the squat-bend ought to be rented by mattress and beer companies as advertising space.

When you get home, you need to pee too urgently to take your clothes off first. You unsnap your coat and hurdle yourself to the toilet, your loosened coat catching on the doorsill and, perhaps, ripping. You are now beginning to feel the new circumference your body occupies. Your arms are so inflated that you can't draw them tightly to yourself; your legs so constrained that despite sitting with your knees wide apart, your thighs touch. Try to change the toilet paper or another task requiring you to reach one arm across yourself. Try to scratch your back. Try to wipe yourself. Feel how narrow your range of motion is when you wash your hands or untie your boots. Take note of the exertion required to do these things. Note the damp places on your body. The small of your back. The secret creases of your groin. Your scalp. Your upper lip. If you take your socks off, they will stiffen from your sweat. The back of the knees of your leggings will be moist. The crotch of your underwear will be as wet as if you'd wet yourself, and the cups of your bra will be fetid with sweat.

Hug someone. Her hands won't meet where they customarily do. and she may not hug you the way she usually does. She may be so confused by your self-presentation that she opts to hold you by the upper arms and buss you instead. Nor, equally sadly, will your arms reach around her. Sit down and try to cross your legs. Pick up a baby or cat or pillow and let it sit in your lap, noting whether it slides off or whether you can nuzzle it comfortably. Sit on a low seat and stand up. You will have to plant your hands on your knees to do this and you may have to rock into the movement to achieve the momentum to accomplish it.

If you want to know more about what it's like to be fat, don this ensemble on a July afternoon. People will look at you and wonder if you're crazy, which is not unlike Gwyneth Paltrow's realization, when she strolled around Tribeca in her *Shallow Hal* fat suit, that "nobody would even make eye contact with me . . . when someone [is] slightly outside what we all consider normal, you think, oh it's polite not to look. But actually, it's incredibly isolating."[59]

If you are fat and want to know what it's like not to have so much weight anchoring you to the ground (this is not for the faint of heart), lift the apron of fat on your belly onto the kitchen counter. Feel the relief in your feet and lower back. Think what you would do if your body always felt that light—where you would walk, how you would dance, the places you could reach.

Then put on a piece of music you're not familiar with—say, Igor Stravinsky's "Circus Polka." Tap your feet to the time, and you'll find the beat shifts away from you, like the shore in a receding wave. As soon as you feel the elephants bending their knees and swaying with the tuba, the trumpets usher in a star turn, not lithe—that belongs to the woodwinds—but deft, certain, and sometimes dancing with the fluty ballerinas.

Stravinsky wrote the polka at the request of George Balanchine, who was the choreographer for the Ringling Brothers Barnum and Bailey Circus in the early forties. Stravinsky agreed to do it only if the elephants were "very young." Did he want the animals smaller or more limber and able to move in counterpoint to the many voices the music speaks in? Would classically trained elephants resist the bursts the polka asks them to dance to?

You are listening to a world. Fifty elephants and fifty beautiful girls parade around the center ring, the elephants' huge feet smacking the sawdust, which forms a faint gauze in the air that is rich with the smell of popcorn and cotton candy. Madoc, the prima pachyderma, tricked out in six-foot pink plumes and a glittering white-and-pink saddle, kicks and bows as her cohorts sway in contrasting rhythm.

---

59 Gwyneth Paltrow, interviewed by Prairie Miller, *NY Rock*, November 2001.

Kids laugh, squeal, cry, whine as the strings pick up the brass section to repeat the music's theme, joining the cymbals two octaves higher than the bass drum. You can feel yourself in the bleachers, astonished at what the elephants can create because, let's face it, as beautiful as the beautiful girls are, as brightly dressed and daringly décolleté, they can't compete with the plumed elephants that outweigh them and outperform them. Any beautiful girl can perform a *pas de bourrée en arrière*. When an elephant does it, the circus has achieved a hybrid of music, dance, and Gothic architecture.

Think of eleven-year-old Wendy hearing symphonic music for the first time. *The Nutcracker Suite* or *Eine Kleine Nachtmusik* would have been as radical to her tender new ears as our polka, duping her as surely as Stravinsky floats a tune and plunges it into a series of six flat notes. Wendy is listening to the world. She may have felt fat when she listened to the records the audiologist suggested, the adagios more graceful and the scherzos more supple than she knew herself to be. She may have felt as dumb as her teachers had told her she was because she didn't know how such music was made, how Mozart heard it in his head before writing it down, or what it takes for violins to sound as sweet and right as her cat's paw. Such music may have made her feel small and weak, as it was so much bigger, older, and tested than she was. It may also have made her feel courageous because she was looking for the story in the massive dark tunnel of this message from beyond her ken.

One day she will move from the E-Z listening classical albums to late-night college radio's twentieth-century music, which she'll have to turn up to hear. It's a choice between eighties soft rock on 860 AM or the Kronos quartet on 88.9 FM, a choice between music or calling Lindsay to cry about Cal. Calling Lindsay will mean going home or sitting in the car outside Five Continents. On and on the choices go, filling the day with the struggle to feel okay, almost okay, loved despite everything we think we are that isn't okay, and the occasional hope that comes from seeing Madoc the Elephant starring in her own show.

SEVEN

October

The Old and the Other
and the Restless

If publishing was searching for a motto, one candidate would be "never let them see you sweat." I am well-schooled, after fifteen years in the business, and know that for an agent this means never letting anyone question your success. For an author, I know from coaching former clients, it means the same, as well as always being excitedly in the middle of a project that is timely and oozing potential.

The number one rule for an author is to be always excitedly in the middle of a project that is timely and oozing potential. In October 2006, I was closer in spirit and lifestyle to dogs than to the author I had inhabited two years earlier—the thin one who was fully immersed in the publishing world. When I left the Bat Cave at ten thirty one gleaming, cool morning, I was in my work uniform: muddy sweatpants, worn-down Crocs, holey thirty-year-old ragg wool sweater speckled with blond, yellow, and brown dog hair, ponytail tucked into a sweaty baseball cap, grime under my nails, glasses clouded by dog kisses. My knickers were in a twist because after I took Daisy,

Hero, Mellie, and Boomer to the dog run, a two-hour gig of throwing balls, being jumped on, and pulling Boomer out of fights by whatever appendage I could hang on to, I had to muster as much of my inner author as possible.

My former publisher was throwing itself an anniversary bash on the Upper West Side that evening. I was about to arm myself to meet my past. It felt as much like a medieval ritual as it sounds. Any number of ghosts could appear, lance and flail at the ready, to reopen old, barely scabbed wounds.

My darling erstwhile editor would be there with all the people I'd worked with on *Passing for Thin* and editors I'd known as an agent. It was quite possible either or both of my former bosses and their associates would show up among the platters of satay and trays of appletinis. The talk show host whose staff hauled me out to L.A. and dismissed me the next day might be mingling with the bestselling authoress of Chubby Chick Lit. And these were the ghosts from one imprint among twenty. Who knew what cousins might show up?

I was going because I know the cardinal rule of this game, in which I still need my former publisher's support, is to make them want me.

The Frances who last made her way to the offices overlooking the Hudson had hair that was perfectly cut and colored, her eyebrows waxed and eyelashes dyed. Her fingernails were the envy of the editorial staff when they passed around the feature about her that ran in *Time* magazine. She had clothes for any occasion, and she was courted and admired by the press and readers. If I no longer had all of these assets in my obesity, at least I knew where to go for the primping. I hoped I could fake everything else.

Over the course of seven months of bouncing in and out of abstinence since March, I'd lost thirty pounds with a lot of lapses along the way. I'd held on to 220 pounds for two months, gaining a little, then re-losing it. Was I afraid of life as it approached two hundred pounds, that threshold of misses' departments and the glow of publishing *Passing for Thin*? I'd begun taking Klonopin, an antianxiety medication in the Valium family, in order to overcome the social anxiety I'd developed in my shrunken world. I went to therapy and to twelve-step meetings as faithfully as I could manage, working on the steps with Patty, my sponsor. That autumn, I invested in some new clothes that were the antithesis of my work duds—velvets, mostly, and satins and pearl-buttoned blouses, in chocolate, deep purple, black, and white. They were 18s and 20s, down two sizes from March, and numbers that felt closer to home.

I made my choices in order to get as far away as possible from dogs and the Bat Cave. Tonight was my debut as thinner, fancier, more sociable than I'd been in a grim long time.

I hurried the dogs home so I could get a quick manicure before picking up another pack. When the afternoon posse was delivered to their doors, I scuttled to have my hair washed and blown out. By the time the door buzzed, I'd gotten halfway through Elvis Costello and Burt Bacharach's *Painted from Memory*, hair and makeup, conservative wool trousers and blazer paired with a sheer blouse showing my prettiest, midnight blue bra.

"Hi," he said, and my heart split in two, one part dropping to the pit of my stomach, the other rising first to my throat and then to my forehead, which always burned in his presence. The night's first ghost, the man who had broken me four years ago, the friend we'd worked hard to save from the lover who stopped loving me, had kindly agreed to squire me, a verb as literal as it was figurative. His "hi" ran a falling scale of four notes and warmed me like caramel, and his face was still always the face that met me on the Metro-North platform, looking up at me from the steel steps, smiling, saying, emphatically, "Yes."

"Hi," I said briskly. "I've been running all day, but I'll be ready in five minutes.

"I know you hate these questions," I went on as he sat down at my computer and started doodling around, "and I know you don't care what women wear, but I'm a wreck, so you're going to have to choose." In one hand, I held out a strand of heavy black Apache tears. In the other was a double loop of filigreed sterling silver with bolts of uncut turquoise.

"That one," he said to the silver. "I don't like big blocky jewelry. Speaking as a guy, of course. So I'm probably wrong."

"Silver it is," I said, and slipped the necklace on and started scratching through earrings for its match.

"You look great, by the way. I can see the difference."

I'd learned several important rules from my first weight loss. One of them is to simply say thank you. Don't defend, don't explain, don't demur. But this was Scott. No one knew me and my last three years better. "I feel like I've just stepped over the boundaries into my real body," I added. "It feels good."

Nothing felt better than his genuine, unsolicited "You look great." As many men as I'd been with since we broke up, no matter that a couple of times I'd lost a bit of my heart to someone, hearing it from Scott was hearing it from someone who'd once flushed at my praise as well.

"'Course," he said, "we hicks from Connecticut don't cotton to women going out nekkid." I grabbed my blazer thanking God I had cover.

At the door, the publisher gushed, "I loved your book!" I smiled at him, a nonanswer that shows my best asset, something Scott had taught me in our salad days of falling in love with the Other Frances. "If he loved it, he could have bought the next one," I whispered to Scott as we inched into the two-story living room with library ladders that could slide around more books than I'd ever possessed, sold, lost, given away, donated, or worn out. It was hot, kaleidoscopic with a hundred people I couldn't separate the faces of, champagne rather than martinis, and spanakopita-crabcakes-dolmades-eggrolls-crostini-shrimp passed by white-coated waiters. Scott fought his way to the seltzer and then I plowed our way to my ex-editor.

My ex-editor, who is so young and fresh that she could be a twelve-year-old, brimmed with excitement to see me, to meet Scott, to hear about his new book. She also brimmed with excitement when she spotted her assistant in another clump of happily boozing youngsters. I admired her professional glitter and let her get back to it as soon as possible, caught by my publicist for a quick hello and by my copy editor, whom I'd not met in person. Scott inspected name tags and gracefully stepped in when I introduced him to these few people and told them about his work. I wanted his handsome and self-assured presence to erase twenty pounds from my aura. It all went pretty quickly, with a couple of perfunctory hors d'oeuvres and our envious perambulation of domesticity on Central Park West, before I turned to Scott and begged, "Can we please leave now?"

Fittingly, because the party was thrown by part of the company that published Truman Capote, we ended up with a bucket of popcorn at *Infamous*. The aptness of our movie choice, made on the basis of what was playing soonest as we walked up Broadway, was mutually squeamish. Scott maintained he would never write his own memoir, which has some nice gory touches to it, while I had, and had done so with little sugarcoating for the major characters in my life, including Scott. It was Truman's year, and the question of the year, in both *Infamous* and *Capote*, was how far he—or any writer—would go to get the best story. Scott and I knew that my answer would be whatever it takes for the story. We left the theater in silence, a wider margin of space between our shoulders than usual. The shelter of the cab brought us closer and when we pulled up at Grand Central, where he'd catch a train back to Connecticut, I kissed him good-bye and said, without thinking—as automatically as the next breath—"I love you."

"I love you, too," he said.

"I'll talk to you in a minute." I hurried the moment on with a wave to how often we spoke on the phone. He slid out of the car, and I craned out to add, "Thanks for walking me through that thing."

"It was fun, hon. I enjoyed it."

A half hour later, Daisy and I walked down Willow Street, past Truman Capote's basement apartment in a yellow brick house I photographed seasonally for its window boxes and red climbing roses. I knew that, unlike that first time I'd told Scott I loved him, there would be no email waiting for me to say that I shouldn't regret the words. "When God hands you a gift, he also hands you a whip," Capote wrote in the preface of *Music for Chameleons*. "And the whip is good for self-flagellation solely."

An important distinction to make in how I regard my bodies lies in the words *old* and *other*. My old body, ten years younger than the one I inhabited in October, verged on circus-freak fat. My "other" body differentiates my thin body as distinct, separate, alien (the imagery I explored in *Passing for Thin*). To say "my other body" is to say I have two bodies, the one I have on and the other one stashed away in closets and bins and air-sealed bags, waiting for the right occasion. While I no longer think of being thin as being alien, I do think of it as being a completely separate entity from the well-padded body I wore to the party. They're all mine but, like shoes, my body now is a well-worn pair of Crocs, whereas my other body is my hand-embossed CYDWOQ heels. My old body is a pair of frayed Keds, worn without shoelaces because my feet are too fat to tie them.

For a fat kid, thin was a cure-all. It would end the teasing. My parents and brothers would love me and be proud of me. I would marry George Harrison. Later, I vaguely thought a simple spin of some dial would reward me with the tweed-coated guy from *Mystery Date* at my door. I'd dance en pointe and play ingénue roles. Later still, I'd wanted a heaping plate of cold revenge on all the people I'd envied for their looks, abilities, and/or successes. A mere glance from the corner of my eye would do it.

Most of all, I wanted being thin to blast depression from my body and my life.

But once we have lost a lifetime's obesity and lived in a thin body, thin is a specific set of signifiers our desires and energies concentrate upon. For me, thin is a suit tailored for me in a Necco wafer brown with a box pleated skirt and short, vaguely military jacket, worn with a boatneck black sweater that has no back. Thin is a pair of velvet

Blackwatch plaid jeans. Thin is having spaces between the joints of my fingers and sore knees from sleeping on my side.

Not long after the publishing party, I had dinner with Pam Peeke. The author of *Body for Life* had taken an interest in me, *Passing for Thin,* and this book. One thing about Pam is that she comes directly and bluntly to the point. "Do you *know* how lucky you are?" she asked in a tone that made me sit back on the banquette and assemble a hasty list (*to be alive, to have a successful book and a new contract, to have an education . . .*) that might answer her question. "*You* gained *half* your weight back!"

I remained slumped away from the table. *Lucky?*

"Statistically, you should have gained it *all* back, and then some. You've beaten the odds!"

I thought about it for a moment, nodded, and returned to my chicken.

"But you gotta stop fuckin' around now. You're fifty, Frances. Time is not on your side."

The riot act had been read. I went home that night thinking about my twitchy weights that made me crazy. Sometimes crazy enough to walk Daisy to the deli for a pint of Ben & Jerry's before bed.

Yes: I'm lucky. I did not return to the circus-freak fat of 338 pounds. I look like a lot of overweight women, a category I can describe by our clothing. In our most well-made, pretty outfits, we look like we are trying *so hard* to fake out spectators that our effort makes our seams look as though they are about to burst. In anything else, we either look as though we're trying to be *au courant* (leggings are in—hurray! Isn't this leopard-spotted blouse cute??) or too much as though we don't care what we're wearing. There are many of us, thankfully. Only once in my second obesity has someone insulted me directly, and I believe she was one of those original *Mayflower* passengers granted the privilege of blunt speech.

I grieve the loss of my other body. I fear my old body more than anything short of the death of my parents. The line at which I cross into my old body is 250 pounds. With such emotionally charged feelings about my weight, why, as Pam put it, was I fuckin' around playing fat arpeggios in the same, eighteen-month-old range of thirty pounds?

There are many reasons I could give, but I think it comes down to the term I use for my body as it is between 200 and 250 pounds: restless. I am so restless to break the barrier of 220 and then 200 pounds that I can't wait. When I do, for a while, and approach the slightly-too-big size 18, I get caught up in some crisis that I eat through, whether it's boarding a difficult dog or visiting my parents or a dip into one of my periodic depressions.

I am too restless to sit still in meetings, read myself to sleep at night, journal my days, stay in the moment. I was restless when I was my other self, too, but it was a restlessness to do and experience, whereas this is a restlessness to be. My old self was rarely restless, consistently anesthetized by carbohydrates into the stillness of a snowwoman.

My old self had an elaborate fantasy life. Parts of it depended on being thin, such as the oncologist husband and our daughter named Maggie, or teaching at a la-di-dah Eastern college and having my hag's fag's baby. I had designs for my literary fame that included a thatched house in the Cotswolds, which I decorated before falling asleep at night. I retreated to Elizabeth and Fitzwilliam Darcy's life after their I-do. (I should have written that last one. I could have led the pack in the continuation of their saga and bought the house in Stow-on-the-Wold.)

Twelve-step Think has a bajillion mottos that stick whether I want them to or not. "One day at a time" destroyed those ongoing fantasies. It's not that I don't want things anymore. Not long after the party, Katie passed on a chain email that asked a lot of personal questions our friends might not know about us. The last question was "What would you like to accomplish/do before you die?" I surprised myself with my answer: "EVERYTHING. Write great books, live in Venice, own a Victorian house, have more dogs, be thin, go to Prague, be in love & be loved back . . ." One difference between my answer to that questionnaire and my old dreams is that I actually make an effort at getting thin and writing. Another difference is that I figure they're all achievable if I keep my eyes on the work at hand. There was never any possibility that I'd wake up next to Mr. Darcy one morning.

For all the fantasies my old self played with after I turned out the light, I had no hope. More precisely, my hope was a child's rubber hammer rather than a chisel. Want is the stepchild of hope: I wanted to write and to be thin, but I didn't hope for them because I had no sustained, finished success with them. In March 2006 when I saw 250 pounds on the greyhounds' scale, I was still in possession of the hope born of success, and I had precise tools with which to carve another self.

I just didn't have the energy to pick up my planner and scorp to whittle away at my cravings.

In the anticlimax of my night of glamour with Scott and with bags of Halloween candy and pumpkin pies filling the shelves of the neighborhood stores, I was in the high state of cravings that comes with cool weather and the expectations of the food pentathlon of the holidays looming ahead. I knew there was another relapse looming. What size would I be when I went to visit my parents at Christmas? Worse, what size would I be when I got back to Brooklyn?

I tend to be a bed-binger, which is uncomfortably close to night-eating disorder.[60] I like to be under the covers with a sedative already twining through my system before I pour on the sugar. I like the

---

60 "The core criterion is an abnormally increased food intake in the evening and night-time, manifested by (1) consumption of at least 25 percent of intake after the evening meal, and/or (2) nocturnal awakenings with ingestions at least twice per week . . . These criteria must be met for a minimum duration of three months." K. C. Allison, et al., "Proposed Diagnostic for Night Eating Syndrome," *International Journal of Eating Disorders*, April 17, 2008. Albert Stunkard, a pioneer in defining this disorder, suggests that wanting high carbohydrates at night increases serotonin levels enough to make sleep easier.

setting because I know I'll be asleep soon, and it's luxurious to be in as close an approximation of the womb as is compatible with food. I eat late at night—a common time for wrong-eaters—because I'm at my loneliest and weakest, because I have no immediate responsibilities to fill, because I survived another day, because I am dissatisfied with the net results of the day, or occasionally because I am pleased and want to celebrate them. Dissatisfaction—regret at having goofed off instead of writing, guilt that I didn't give the dogs enough playtime, anger that I didn't do simple chores—is the worst demon in the bunch. I eat before sleep to forget I was fatuously awake.

A typical bedtime "snack" for me could be a box of Honey Bunches of Oats, milk, and Entenmann's chocolate doughnuts—4,400 calories—or a pint of Ben & Jerry's chocolate chip cookie dough ice cream and a twelve-pack of Oreo Cakesters—2,580 calories. You can understand my dismay, then, when I looked up the definition of a binge, a recent addition to the classes of eating disorders. Specialists are vague about fixing on a precise definition, but the Mayo Clinic says,

> When you have binge-eating disorder, sometimes called compulsive overeating, you regularly eat excessive amounts of food (binge). A binge is considered eating a larger amount of food than most people would eat under similar situations. For instance, you may eat 10,000 to 20,000 calories worth of food during a binge, while someone following a normal diet may eat 1,500 to 3,000 calories in a day . . . A binge episode is typically considered to last about two hours. But the duration also is under debate, and some experts say binges can last an entire day.[61]

---

61 Mayo Clinic Staff, "Binge Eating Disorder Symptoms," April 20, 2009, http://www .mayoclinic.com/health/binge-eating-disorder/DS00608/DSECTION=symptoms (accessed).

Two hours? Ten *thousand* calories? I graze in my parents' house, often in the middle of the night when I wake up and can't get back to sleep, edging closer to being an official night-eater, but I can't honestly remember purposefully assembling the food necessary to eat for two hours.

The Mayo Clinic and other eating-disorder clinics gloss over the emotional and physical damage caused by my measly four thousand calories or Lindsay's low-fat craze in her twenties when she'd chomp a couple of cups of dry Grape-Nuts through the night for an 832-calorie well of shame and weight gain. When I walk down Montague Street, I am sure their definitions are too stringent when they claim that anorexia nervosa and bulimia are the most common expressions of eating disorders. I may sleep like the (sweaty) dead after my ice cream and cookies, but I wake to shame, self-punishing soliloquies, no taste for my ritual coffee and cigarettes, increased hunger through the day, and diarrhea. Even eating abstinent food in too much quantity at the wrong time produces those feelings and physical reactions.

"I still haven't decided if I'm a food addict or just fucked up," Lindsay said in IM one morning. *Everyone is a food addict*, I thought to myself. It's biological necessity.

Twelve-step-ese, with its extensive nomenclature, can distort one's identity. We introduce ourselves, according to the kind of meeting we're at, as "compulsive overeaters," "compulsive eaters," or "food addicts." Sometimes we preface our statement with the words "I'm a gratefully recovering [food addict/compulsive overeater]." I have the First Compulsive Bite discussion with Patty at least once a month. The FCB, as I've noted earlier, is the demarcation between abstinence and relapse. But when I'm hungry (and hunger feels like a terminal illness to me), *every* bite, weighed, measured, without sugar or flour, is compulsive, not to mention savage. "Can we change that to the First Compulsive Bite *after* we've eaten what we're supposed to?" I ask.

Even after all these years in the Rooms, the jargon still irks me.

"Hey! How are you? Are you abstinent?" a friend will ask after not seeing me in a while. *No*, I'm aching to say. *I'm Frances*. "At least you're abstinent!" Patty said the day I sobbed that the state demanded another five hundred dollars that I didn't have. That was certainly a comfort.

When Lindsay wondered whether she was a food addict, I realized that when I raise my hand I may use the meeting's going jargon—a food addict or compulsive overeater—but I add that I am a sugar addict. I'm also a starch/fats/protein addict, but at some point I have to shut up.

In the course of two months, Katie's one piece of dark chocolate a day had turned into a cinnamon toast mania, and by October she had regained twenty pounds, seven less than she'd started out at in June. When I inevitably bought a box of orange-frosted cupcakes, I hated myself for being relieved that we were in the same boat. A woman on a needed diet often avoids women who need to diet and aren't doing so. Free eating is infectious because we envy it, even when we are flush with success and excitement. Katie and I avoided each other when we weren't in sync, but she was the only one who understood a twelve-stepper's steep hill and no brakes when it came to alternating sugar and fasting.

"Do you think I can get abstinent?" I pleaded from under the covers of my bed, scratching Daisy's butt as she hunkered tightly against me.

"Do you think *I* will?" she countered.

"Yes," I said staunchly. "Something's going to bottom out, and you'll go back to Program."

"What if I don't bottom out? I mean, I weigh 420 pounds. I can't go anywhere or do anything. What's it going to take?"

"Getting really, really tired of food or not being able to do stuff. Getting tired of belonging to food instead of yourself. I don't know."

"God, yes, that's so right: belonging to food. Me and my food. We're a club."

"Me, too," I said. I reached down to stroke Daisy's ears and she shifted away from me. I felt like my club had just been reduced. "I gotta start going to meetings, but I'm so tired all the time."

"I frigging hate meetings," Katie said in an exhalation of something pent up. "I hate walking in all fat and gross-looking, and seeing people I knew from before."

"It's not your fault. You're a compulsive overeater. It's what you *do*. It could be any one of them in a year."

"Except it's now, and it's not them who are fat. It's me and I can't stop."

"I know," I said softly. "Me, either." The clock read ten. It wasn't that cold outside and Gristedes was still open. If I had vanilla Oreos and ice cream, I'd sleep well. If Katie got to, why couldn't I?

"Get abstinent, Frances. I need you to. I need to see a success I like for a change."

Despite the seasonal lapse, I held on to that 220 pounds. But seven months after seeing 250 on the scale, I hadn't lost the weight I should have. I knew exactly what to do, and yet I didn't do it consistently and rigorously enough. It was a double failure, this maintenance of regained fat. What was the point of trying when I was so pointless myself?

The hundred-pound gain was disappointment on a grand scale. The list goes on and on: a hundred pounds, for God's sake: *ten* clothing sizes in the extremely limited storage space of the Bat Cave! Should I have left publishing, or was I cut out for it in the first place? There was the novel I wanted to write and didn't, and the man who could have come to love me whom I broke up with for Scott. It was depressing, but I'm coming to believe that depression—and compulsive eating— are fraternal twins and just as dodgy as my old fantasy life. Food and depression isolate me, keep me as self-bound and self-preoccupied as fantasy did. Each, if I'm not careful, is the black hole of futility at the end of the day. What's the difference between spending an evening making up a story about spending a winter in Venice, and digging a pit with my failures and insufficiencies and filling it with ice cream?

Neither is reality. Neither is constructive. Neither qualifies as being aware and connected.

Five mostly abstinent years and a loss of 188 pounds means I'll never really leave the Rooms. They work too well to leave forever because they operate on a rock bottom of truth and honesty. I *did* hurt people by my compulsive eating; I have character flaws to enumerate and work on that I carried into my other life. The danger of my tether to the Rooms was that there was no need to rush because sooner or later I'd be desperate, return to the meetings, my food plan, being answerable to a sponsor and to the steps. You can't go off to Sugarland when you've been in a twelve-step program without taking the knowledge with you that you're a compulsive overeater and food addict, for which you have found only one treatment.

Seven months earlier, in the greyhounds' bathroom, I *knew* that I had to lose the hundred pounds. My old self wanted to lose weight, but it wasn't an inviolable certitude. In my restlessness, my capacity to hope, decide, commit, dare, try, stretch, change, achieve is tied to the food plan that I lose weight on. I wanted my sanity more than whatever looks I possessed, and I wanted to reclaim my victory over my worst enemies, foremost among them, my compulsion and myself.

Hope, the antecedent of intention and action, kept me from giving my thin clothes away. My friend B.J. has not gotten rid of her thin clothes, either, but neither has she put any effort or expression into the size she wears now. In fact, she's adamant on the subject. "I won't spend serious money until I'm 135 pounds," she says. B.J. works outdoors, so she, too, trash-dresses. I haven't seen her when she's not working, but I assume she makes do with a uniform of black pants, a big white shirt, and slightly scary boots. The glamour I want from velvet she claims by wearing her sunflower-sized diamond stud earrings pretty much 24/7.

Katie kept her thin clothes until deciding to remedy some of her financial distress by selling them online. ("Gently used" is the code for shoes and clothes that didn't make it beyond a season. "Gently used" when we were thin and didn't perspire so much or so rankly, when we didn't spill salad dressing on our bosoms, when we didn't wear out the thighs of trousers and the soles of our shoes.) She said that those clothes belong to a different Katie, perhaps not other, as I think of myself wearing 8s and 10s, but a past Katie, a Katie she wants to change (to harden, to love), work she continued as she struggled to stick to her food plan.

I decided to let the matter of my other clothes go until I fit into them. Like Katie, I was working hard to shore up weaknesses that contributed to my relapse. I wouldn't be the other Frances or, if I could help it, this restless Frances. I hoped to fit into those clothes one day, but the question was whether they would fit *me*.

It came quickly to pass that Scott called me while I was spending the holidays with my parents in Arizona to wish me a happy New Year. In the course of telling me he saw *Charlotte's Web* on Christmas, he mentioned that Sarah came down on Boxing Day.

I let a beat pass. "That sounds nice," I said calmly, and let the conversation go where Scott wanted—to his freelance PR gigs and his crazy bosses, my parents' health, or the exploits of his kitten. I was barely there, sick at heart, and burning with curiosity. Fifteen minutes later, in a lull of chat, I said, "So. Who's Sarah?"

He cleared his throat. His unease about where to start was as tangible as the ceramic handle on my coffee mug. "We met through my blog," he said. "We've been writing and talking for a while. You'd like her."

"I'm sure I would," I lied through my clenched teeth. "Is it serious?"

He laughed. "You know me. I don't know where I'll be next summer. She lives in upstate New York and she's busy and I'm busy. It has its complications. But we seem to have a thing, and obviously, I wouldn't mention it if I didn't think you should know about her."

Ah. The old "there's something I need to talk to you about" speech. He had relied on me to circle the conversation back to her, making me look as possessive and jealous as I felt and wanted to hide. I didn't know whether to think him a coward or brave, finally, for telling me. *He must be falling in love,* I thought, *and I must be important to him if he's calling me the day after she left.* My heart took a slow stroll to my throat, like a snowball working its way uphill and gathering more snow as it went.

"I'm glad for you. You deserve—the best."

"Thank you," he said quietly.

"I have to admit, though, that I—" My voice faltered. I took a breath and bit my lips between my teeth. "I guess I hoped we'd get it together sometime. You and me." I laughed. Harshly, for his benefit. *You're off the hook, Scott: I won't make a scene.* "I fail to understand why you're not madly in love with me."

He laughed, too, more warmly. "It's one of those things you can't explain, hon."

Hon. Oh, the stupidity of men.

"I know. It's not like I haven't been in love with other men in the last five years." I'd had crushes and affairs in that time, some of them serious, most of them with many extra pounds. Another thing I'd brought from my other self was the knowledge of how to flirt and that, in middle age, while thin is nice, it's not essential for every, or even, most men. "I just kept kind of coming back to you."

"Like I said, Frances, I don't know what I'm doing. But this is good now."

"I'll adjust," I said, wondering how I could bear this news, the ache in my throat that was assuming the hugeness of a love that had survived other loves, a love that had survived as much punishment as I'd hurled at myself in the last three years. "We'll talk when I get back to New York. I'm a blob when I'm with Mom and Dad."

We did talk, Scott and I, desultorily, from time to time. I let him do the calling; I answered emails and sent the occasional joke or political analysis along, but I didn't initiate contact. In the spring, he called to share the news of a job offer and in the conversation mentioned he was coming down with Sarah's cold.

They'd been together longer than he and I had. I reached out and kneaded Daisy's ears. Without waking, she shifted and rolled onto her back for a tummy rub, legs akimbo, profoundly trusting. "So things are . . . good . . ." I put out tentatively.

"Yeah," he said. "It's been a tough time financially. She's made it better than it would have been."

"Good."

I answered his questions, offering little information or news of my own. We said good-bye quietly. Later I emailed Mimi, Wendy, and Lindsay, whose boy troubles are a common denominator Katie didn't share at the time, that I had to tell Scott we couldn't be friends. One by one, each called to offer support and assurance. I wrote a loving farewell email and received one in return. After nearly six years it was over. Only an impotent ache survived the loss of the man who had become a best friend, my dim flickering expectation that we would be more than friends, the survivals of breakups he'd put me through, and a hundred lesser demons loosed from the well in my heart.

But I was also proud of having finally cut the ties between Scott and me, something I'd needed to do for years. Thin or fat, I'd helplessly allowed the feeble candle of Scott to go on burning. Something was shifting.

One chilly cornflower blue morning that October, I chucked my backpack and leashes on a bench in the dog run and started throwing balls.

It was more work throwing balls for Henry than for Daisy, even though Daisy yapped constantly for the next toss. Henry's attention span was such that he tended to drop his ball as he meandered back, which meant I then had to go find it. I took satisfaction in doing a physical job at fifty years of age. The experience of having been thin gave me the confidence to get up every morning and collect these magnificent beasts, walking them one-handed as I smoked a cigarette and steered them out of people's way, dividing the world into dog friendly and dog phobic with a radar that became second nature.

I learned a lot about humans from the dogs, and I've learned that the stupidest humans are other dog owners.

A very lovely blonde woman with several preadolescent daughters came into the park with a bouncing blonde golden doodle—that year's It Dog, half golden retriever, half standard American poodle. With the golden's affability and gentleness, and the poodle's intelligence and lack of shedding, they've become popular with families.

"This is Macomber," one of the girls said breathlessly as they all sat down on the bench where my stuff was stowed. "He's five months old, and we're meeting his littermate to play!"

Daisy was screeching for her ball, and Henry was winding in and out of my legs. "That's nice," I said, not really understanding her high-pitched, excited rush of words. Henry took one look at Macomber and sprang at him, ecstatic to make a new friend who was also a puppy, with a puppy's sloppy energy. Macomber concurred and rolled over on his back as Henry darted around and over him, biting his neck.

"Henry's a little necky," I told the mom. "I can get him off if you don't like it."

"We'll see what happens," she said. I smiled and turned back to Daisy's hopping, glass-breaking demands. A moment later, I saw that Macomber was stuck under low-slung Henry, who was gnawing the doodle's collar.

"Henry!" I yelled, a futile gesture. Henry no more came when called than he balanced his checkbook. I reached out and hauled him off Macomber, who promptly took off after a play bow invitation for Henry to chase him.

Chase and catch—and go back to biting at his neck. Once again I hauled him off and this time Mom called Macomber onto the bench, where he sat on my backpack as she soothed him.

"I think your dog's too rough," she said.

"I'll get him busy with the ball," I answered, and lofted Henry's favorite red Cuz to entice him out into the park. Out of the corner of my eye, I noticed another party of young moms and kids entering the double gate at the top of the hill. Macomber's littermate bounded down, followed by Charles, a black flat-coated retriever that lives down the block from us. Henry perked up at so much puppy energy and went back to wrestling.

This time Mom got hysterical. "Pull him off! Pull him off!" she cried from the bench she was now standing on. I was grabbing for Henry's collar as he did his Mohammad Ali dance-like-a-butterfly-and-sting-like-a-bee routine. I needed another five or eight seconds to get hold of him successfully when she threw her coffee cup and hit Henry on the head.

Henry is a big baby. If a dog barks or nips at him, he cries and runs away. Had the wrestling match gone on any longer, he would have taken his turn on his back as the others went for *his* neck. There wasn't a mean bone in his body, and next to the sixteen-year-old Lab that I walked in the afternoon, he was the dog I was least scared of being on the streets with. I didn't expect the woman to know that, but throwing a cup of coffee—?

I pulled Henry away and turned to her as she climbed down to reclaim Macomber, who was shaking himself and waiting for Henry to take his next shot. I took one step up to her so that we were chest-to-chest, our faces two inches apart.

"Don't you *ever* fucking hit a dog," I yelled, jabbing my right index finger in the narrow space between us. "You want to hit a dog; you hit *me*. But don't you *ever* fucking hit a dog. Do you understand?"

I stepped back and grabbed Henry's collar again and walked him over to leash him. The woman half giggled to her friends, "I'm just surprised I hit him!"

I wasn't surprised the next morning that I'd had a night of Zoloft-vivid dreams about Alix.

Don't you ever *fucking hit a dog.*

Words I should have said to Alix.

When I told Patty, my sponsor, about the incident and the dreams, she studied her hands in her lap, and said, sadly, "We spend our lives trying to learn to protect the kid we once were."

"I seem to be playing out my dramas through my dogs," I said. We were sitting in front of the Supreme Court trying to catch the last autumn warmth. Downwind from the farmers' market, the smell of coffee and moldering leaves, apples and basil and all the good things from the earth washed over us. "The problem is trying to learn," I answered. "If I could learn, I might have a chance of finishing the job."

"You're getting more aware," she said, and reached over to hold my hand. "That's a gift."

After eight years, I was more aware of what propelled me to eat. Part of controlling my disease is living with my dis-ease as I parse and mend it. I had protected Henry the way I should I have protected myself. I was proud of that. I thought it was an epiphany of sorts.

Perhaps it was. But reenacting one drama leaves so many others waiting their turn.

A week later I was trying to take a photo of the leaves piling up on a stoop across the street. Daisy was tossing a stick around, making the pictures blur until she settled at my feet to chew it. I had finally gotten a clear shot—no tugging on the leash, no traffic in the way—when suddenly she reared up from the sidewalk and jumped on a man, barking frantically. "Daisy!" I yelled, startled, my heart pounding. I pulled her off and yanked us both back a couple of steps.

"Does your dog always attack people?" He nodded toward the police notice about no parking that was taped to the post my shoulder had been twelve inches from as I took pictures. Daisy had been between me and the post. "I wanted to read the sign."

"I'm sorry," I said, "you scared her."

"Oh, no, you don't," he said, his voice rising. "Don't you put the blame on me. You should be apologizing, not blaming!"

"I'm sorry, sir." My own voice was coming from somewhere behind me, controlled, level, quiet. "I did apologize. I just wanted to explain *why* she jumped at you. She was scared."

"Now I know why your dog is crazy," he yelled.

"I'm sorry," my voice said. "She's a *dog*. She was scared."

"Fuck you, woman. *Fuck. You.*"

"I'm *sorry*. She's just a dog. She's a *dog*. She gets scared. Don't you understand?"

He had backed up some ten feet and was fumbling at his pocket. Was he going to call 911 or take a cell phone picture of us to post around the neighborhood? In the second it took me to question what he was doing, he whipped around and stomped down the steps to the apartment building he was in front of and disappeared.

I fell apart. We'd been on our way to do an errand, but halfway down the next block, Daisy stopped to sit on a stoop as I sobbed. She looked at me with her intelligent, enigmatic amber eyes. I reached out and scrunched up the loose skin of her neck to rub her. "You're a dog," I whispered, and sniffed. "You were scared. Couldn't he understand?"

My reaction was not, of course, entirely about Daisy. Couldn't Scott understand how much I hurt during the pre-breakups that became re-breakups, the casual mentions of his new love—even the sound of his voice?

Couldn't all the ghosts understand how scared I was? How alone?

Apparently not. I hadn't had the words to explain and they (Scott, Alix, my family) probably hadn't had the ears to hear.

In the end, it doesn't matter what's behind my compulsion to overeat. That's the hardest truth I carried with me as I ate myself a hundred pounds heavier.

I ate for two days after the incident with Daisy. Cookies, cake, ice cream, bread—and then more yet. My belly button wept from the volume. I slept heavily between bouts, accomplishing almost nothing, dreading waking up and still being too full to eat. I talked about the incidents with Henry and Daisy with the AFGs and with friends. I wasn't searching for reassurance or love in sugar. It was oblivion I wanted, stilling my own voice, my history. *Don't hit me. I'm scared. Don't you understand?* But then I would wake up to another voice in the stew. *I disgust myself.*

I knew what to do: make phone calls to people in the Rooms, write about it, pray over it, call Patty sixty times if I had to. But I didn't. I willfully remained alone, thinking I should have shrugged it all off, wondering how other people let go of unpleasant interactions. I felt foolish and infantile, and I didn't want to be a burden to my friends.

I will never be able to binge with the impunity I had in 1998—or in 2003 or in late October of 2006. I know too much. I've replayed my long-held dramas, spoken the words of protection and explanation about my dogs that are as much about me, and learned that the words are only important to me—important, horrifying, essential, and pointless if I'm not awake and functioning to move to the next unsaid words and the next clean day, all the way to the happy ending I owe us all.

EIGHT

November

Diets, Food Plans, Pills, and Treadmills

November was sobbing rain, the water falling down the diner windows in waves. Wendy sat across from Mark—the Invisible Man, her August boyfriend—and let out a ragged breath. She could feel her face turning red in blotches, the unfortunate fate of very fair redheads who are determined to hold it together during a breakup scene.

"Please try to understand," Mark said. He slid out of his side of the booth and sat down next to her. "I'm working seventy-two hours a week and trying to see my kids whenever I can. On top of that, it's an hour's drive to your place. My life is too complicated to be involved with anyone right now."

"Does 'It's not you, it's me' come next?" she croaked.

"It *is* me." He put his arm around her shoulder and pulled her into him. "If things were different, I might be able to have a relationship." Wendy's shoulders were shaking, the first sob about to crest. "I can't juggle this many plates. I've tried and I can't. It's not fair to you."

That did it. Wendy grabbed a wad of napkins and began to cry. Loudly.

"Oh, honey . . ." Mark said helplessly.

Do all men work from the same script? She dropped her napkins on the scrambled eggs, grabbed another handful, and blew her nose. Loudly.

"Would you excuse me?" she said. As always, she was pleased that she could slide out of a booth without lurching and without a grease stain in the shape of a half piece of buttered toast on her chest. Still crying, silently now, she walked out of the diner and headed toward home.

Despite the tears running down her face, she could feel her dignity pulsing like a well-used muscle. Wendy Harriet Wicks, formerly 342 pounds, once stuck solidly in a Red Lobster chair, could now leave a booth, leave her eggs and sausage, leave a man to his clichés, and walk home.

At that, she started sobbing again. Eighty pounds lighter, and she still couldn't keep a man. She cried harder when Mark pulled up beside her, opened the passenger door, and held out a four-inch stack of napkins.

They talked all afternoon, and Wendy was ravenous by the time Mark left for Fredericksburg. She had nothing ready to eat in the house except for a box of one-hundred-calorie bags of Doritos and another of fudge-striped cookies, and one can of refried beans. Wendy had some juggling of her own to do.

Were the beans a vegetable, starch, or protein? She had instituted a half-plate rule: one side vegetables, the other side protein and starch.

Tomorrow was Monday. What would she take to work for lunch?

Mark was not the love of her life, but it had been a long haul and a lot of first dates between Cal and the next boyfriend. And oh, how she longed for a boyfriend.

Mark wanted to be friends. He still wanted to go to her cousin's Thanksgiving family reunion with her as they had planned. It would be an overnight trip to Pulaski, a five-hour drive west, and they would be sharing a motel room. Would they have sex? Why would he still want to be her date?

As puffy-eyed and drained as she was, Wendy pulled on a pair of sneakers and drove to Five Continents. Yogurt, Diet Coke, tomatoes, apples, salad bar, rotisserie chicken: she figured that should see her through the next couple of days.

She came home with the Diet Coke and a sizable chunk of imported Cheddar cheese.

Refried beans are a vegetable, she decided. And they were fat free. With one tiny bag of nachos and not even two ounces of the strong cheese, she'd be well under her Weight Watchers points for the day.

If only Mark had been there to take away the cheese and the other six bags of nachos.

Lindsay, Mimi, and Wendy are all on Weight Watchers' Flex Plan, which assigns a point value, calculated by fat, fiber, and calories, for every serving of food found in the continental United States. "There's no need to give up your favorite foods," according to the description of this option, although how *much* an individual can eat is based on gender (and lactation), age, height, weight, activity level, and how many extra "points" are left for the week.

Of course, the promise of having my cake and eating it, too, prompted me to calculate my daily points (including the averaged five of thirty-five weekly Flex Points). Thus that slice of thin-crust pizza topped with vegetables, featured on their website and in their introductory material, would be about one-sixth of my day's food allotment.

Wendy's dinner of three one-hundred-calorie bags of nacho Doritos, refried beans, and what came suspiciously close to six ounces of cheese came to six, three, and sixteen points, respectively. "I overdid it," she told me the next day when she called, sad and defeated over the Invisible Man, "but considering what I *wanted* to eat and didn't, I'll take some success there."

I wish I could point my finger at Wendy but I can't. As long as I've known her, she hasn't finished a night with the incalculable number of points contained in an entire box of Honey Bunches of Oats (1,820 calories), the better part of a quart of skim milk (320 calories), and an eight-pack of Entenmann's frosted devil's food doughnuts (2,480 calories). I wish I could say the same for me.

Americans *love* diets. In June 2007, based on the recommendations of nutritionists and diet experts, *Consumer Reports* ranked the best diet plans and books in the following order:

1. Barbara J. Rolls's *The Volumetrics Eating Plan*
2. Weight Watchers in a near tie with . . .
3. Jenny Craig
4. Slim-Fast
5. eDiets
6. Barry Sears's men's diet from *The Zone*
7. Dean Ornish's *Eat More, Weigh Less*
8. Atkins Diet

In 2004, *Medical News Daily* didn't weigh the top diets of the year, but selected the eight most popular:

1. Atkins Diet
2. Barry Sears's *The Zone*
3. Nicholas Perricone's *The Perricone Prescription*
4. Weight Watchers
5. Dean Ornish's *Eat More, Weigh Less*
6. Macrobiotics
7. Raw foods

Of these eleven diet plans, Lindsay, Katie, Wendy, Mimi, and I have tried about a third. We are underrepresented in these canons because there are an infinite number of diets on the shelves, in store-fronts, on the Internet, on the covers of magazines, in hospitals and workshops and church basements. Because *Consumer Reports* and *Medical News Daily* have listed eleven popular diets doesn't mean that those other methods are always ineffective or unhealthy.

Women who have struggled with their weight and have had suc-cess with weight loss tend to revert to the tried and true.

Which is not to say we haven't been unfaithful to our successes. This is a list, by name or type, of the diets Lindsay, Katie, Wendy, Mimi, and I have tried in the past:

Atkins (Mimi)

Bulimia: vomiting (Katie), laxatives (Frances)

The Diet Center (Frances)

The Food Pyramid (Lindsay)

The Grapefruit Diet (Mimi)

Jenny Craig (Katie)

Low-carb, low-fat, calorie counting (all of us)

The Kay Sheppard Food Plan (Frances and Katie)

Bob Greene and Oprah Winfrey's *Make the Connection*
   (Lindsay)

Medical fasts (Frances and Mimi)

Nutritionist (Mimi)

Nutrisystem (Frances and Mimi)

Over-the-counter weight-loss abettors: Ayds (Wendy)

Prescription drugs: Phen-fen and Redux (Francc and Mimi);
   Eskatrol (Wendy)

The Rice Diet (Lindsay, for one day)

Richard Simmons's Food Mover (Lindsay's only infomercial
   purchase)

Rigid exercise program (Frances and Lindsay)

The Scarsdale Diet (Katie and Mimi)

Self-imposed daytime starvation (all of us)
Slim-Fast and other liquid meal replacements (Frances and
    Wendy)
The South Beach Diet (Wendy)
Twelve-step programs (Frances, Katie, and Wendy)
Mehmet Oz and Michael Roizin's *You: On a Diet* (Katie)
Weight Watchers (Katie, Mimi, Lindsay, and Wendy)

Few of these diets failed. To one degree or another, it was we who failed the diets. In making yet another honest effort to lose weight, we've had to grapple with what parameters we can work within and those that are too difficult, too easy, too self-destructive, or too expensive for our lives and the severity of our tendency toward violence with food.

Lindsay gained weight on her low-fat regimen, eating dry cereal by the handfuls and pasta by the bucket, and one of my ex-sisters-in-law turns orange every few years when she turns to carrots as an alternative to more caloric eating compulsions.

The AFGs' expectations of Thanksgiving ranged from the usual, Lindsay and Jalen would take salad to her parents' house in Akron, to the eclectic, Mimi and I had potlucks for the unfamilied we always attended, for which she always made her family's traditional sweet potato and apple casserole and I had decided to make Paul Prudhomme's sweet-potato pecan pie. I was obviously not planning an abstinent Thanksgiving and had only weak hopes that I'd get enough clean days in the next three weeks that my father wouldn't greet me with a comment or a knowing squeeze of my back fat when he hugged me hello.[62]

Katie's Thanksgiving was foisted on her. Her mother had announced

---

62 According to Health Management Resources, the average Thanksgiving Day meal is a mind-boggling 5,830 calories, February 25, 2009, http://www.hmrprogram.com/documents/ Holiday_dinner.pdf.

that she wanted no visitors and that dinner would be at the country club.

"This is *sooo* deliberate," she hissed when I called after reading about the latest family feud on her blog. "Stephen's wife is mad at me because I couldn't babysit Lily and Nicholas last month when her mother was in the hospital. So I have no place to stay and Mom's banking on me being too ashamed to be seen at the club."

"Hoity-toity," I said.

"But my brother Michael is coming down from Portland with Annie and the girls. They're staying at Stephen's house. So do I drive five hours for dried-out turkey and Pam glaring at me, or do I go to my grandma's?"

"I'd take Grandma for two hundred dollars."

"Which is fine except then there will be a million questions. My niece, Zoë, called me last night. 'We're goin' on the pane, Auntie Kay. Will you come play with us?' She wouldn't stop begging until I told her I had to work so I can send her and Hailey Christmas presents."

"Yiii," I breathed. What could I say?

"Oh, and I'm purging, Frances," she went on as though talking about playing Wednesday-night bridge or doing counted cross stitch. "Do you know what it's like to throw up when you weigh more than four hundred pounds? My back is killing me, and God knows what it's doing to my heart and blood pressure."

"God, Katie, stop. Please?" I could attest to how a box or even a double dose of Ex-lax can limit life. It's painful, humiliating, dehydrating, and sets off a bout of irritable bowel syndrome.

Wendy, despite the women in her family's country cooking, was resolved to not eat at all. It seemed easier than just a bite.

Medically supervised starvation is another risk we've taken and suffered the consequences of. Mimi went through five rounds of protein-sparing modified fasts through Dicken-Harriman Hospital. "I love to eat, I love the texture and taste of food, and hated the horrible sludge that we had to drink instead," she recalls. "It was hard to be social, it was hard to not eat, it was hard to have my hair fall out and my bowels cramp. It was also wicked expensive. Mostly it was weird."

I've done two medical fasts, at St. Luke's and Mount Sinai hospitals in New York City. The protein drinks had to be made in a blender with ice in order to be barely palatable, and while I lost weight rapidly, my weekly blood tests showed my cholesterol was at high risk levels. I found it odd that the St. Luke's doctor made no comment on it.

My father grunted when I read him my blood test results. "How's your breath?"

My breath? I held my hand in front of my mouth and exhaled. Ugh.

"Like a charnel house."

"Ketoacidosis."

Daddy enjoys swinging around medical terms that I won't possibly understand. "Don't you mean supercalifragilisticexpialidocious?"

"I mean you're eating your own body, honey. You're existing on your fat, which is being released into your blood in order to feed your cells. It's too bad you're not protesting something. If you're going to starve, you might as well try to end a war."

I *was* trying to end a war, the one I had with my body. But for the three months of drinking chalk, my mind was full of what I would eat when the fast was over. (Pizza after St. Luke's; prime rib and about a pint of sour cream on a football-sized potato after Mount Sinai.)

My doctor seemed to appreciate Dad's information, saying he hadn't given it much thought. I should have wondered what, exactly, doctors knew, in the early 1990s, about obesity. Wasn't anybody comparing lipids, investigating how the two heads of Janus connect?

The principles underlying extreme dieting are rapid success and simplicity: either don't eat, or eat anything and get rid of it. The common denominator between it and the more reasonable plans the five Angry Fat Girls have succeeded with is simplicity. In looking over the *Consumer Reports* and *Medical News Daily* lists, I'm struck by how much research and expense a follower of some of the other plans has to go to. Ornish and Perricone have each published eight books and Barbara Rolls has two Volumetric books to her credit.

If you want to be overwhelmed, try researching the Atkins diet. Robert Atkins published over a dozen low-carb guides and the Atkins Health and Medical Information Service has followed up with numerous others.

For each plan, there are cookbooks and journals, Internet bulletin boards and chat rooms, branded products and special services, making them as expensive as a hospital fast or the diet groups, each of which has its own books, products, and services. Cooking can be complicated, especially in a family where not everyone is participating. The Zone has come up with a solution. The Zone Seattle, for instance, will, for twelve hundred dollars a month, deliver three meals and two snacks to your door each day, removing the sticky problem of choosing what Zone recipe to make that will also feed your eight-year-old.

This explains some of the popularity of Nutrisystem (which delivers fix-yourself meals for around three hundred dollars a month), the Diet Center (based on lots of supplements, "fat burning appetite suppressing thermogenics," and à la carte meal makings for which an entrée is about two dollars per serving), and Weight Watchers (which has gone in for snacky stuff available at the grocery store and a tie-in deal with Applebee's).

None of the Angry Fat Girls is rolling in money, nor do we have excess time for intense shopping, preparation, appointments, or research.

One day, a fellow blogger, Cherry, was considering going out to buy Bob Greene's new book. Instead, she decided to make a list of all the diet "loot" (books and DVDs) she has around the house, exclusive of specialty diet cookbooks. This is what she came up with.

Prevention Total Body Guide by Selene Yeager ($9.99)
Definition by Joyce L. Vedral PhD ($14.99)
The Pilates Body by Brooke Siler ($18.00)

The 30 Day Total Health Makeover by Marilu Henner ($22.00)

Body for Life by Bill Phillips and Michael D'Orso ($26.95)

Body for Life Success Journal by Bill Phillips ($25.95)

Cliff Sheats' Lean Bodies by Cliff Sheats, Maggie Greenwood-Robinson, and Linda Thornbrugh ($24.95)

The Ultimate New York Body Plan by David Kirsh ($21.95)

The Ultimate Weight Solution by Dr. Phil McGraw ($26.00)

The Biggest Loser by The Biggest Loser Experts and Cast ($18.95)

Protein Power by Michael R. and Mary Dan Eades ($14.95)

Win the Fat War by Anne Alexander ($7.00)

The Thyroid Diet by Mary J. Shomon ($14.95)

Thin for Life by Anne M. Fletcher ($15.00)

The Solution by Laurel Mellin ($10.95)

Just My Size Yoga with Megan Garcia ($14.98)

Yoga Zone Introduction to Yoga by Alan Finger and Al Bingham ($15.30)

Yoga for Weight Loss by Bharat Thakur ($14.98)

Pilates Beginning Mat Workout by Ana Caban ($14.98)—jury still out on this one (in other words, I haven't opened the cellophane on it yet)

Personal Training System with Denise Austin ($14.98)

Prevention Fitness System: Personal Training ($14.98)

The Biggest Loser: The Workout ($14.98)

Billy's Bootcamp ($19.98)

Ultimate Burn & Firm with Kathy Smith ($29.98)

Sound Mind, Sound Body by David Kirsch ($24.95)

Yoga Conditioning for Weight Loss ($14.98)

Cherry's library isn't special, but she is for having broken it down:

Total $ 452.35
Total Weight Lost to Date: 24.4 pounds
Price Per Pound Lost: $18.54

And so, not having the patience to learn ourselves into a Pilates body, and having tried other methods and found ourselves ill, gaining weight, or white-knuckling, we've settled on what is familiar.

The *Consumer Reports* panel says that familiarity does not breed contempt: "Since variety stimulates the appetite, the more monotonous your diet, the less you'll eat."[63] Some experts recommend that dieters have stock meals twice a day and vary the menu for the third.[64] I nodded when I read that. I eat from one of four grains at breakfast and almost always the same lunch.[65] I have seen this in Lindsay, Mimi, and Katie's menus, too. Breakfast and lunch are "deadline" meals, with obligations looming. Lindsay and Mimi often pack their lunches, which have limitations that encourage repetition. Lindsay and Jalen trade off cooking dinner, while Mimi and I shop and cook in volume over the weekend. Our dinners are often the same thing several nights running.

Mimi was the blogging cook among us. Her recipe for Crock-Pot steel-cut oats has gotten the most hits of any topic she has posted (more than four thousand in its first ten months).[66] When Mimi blogs about her Sundays in the kitchen, I'm tempted to propose marriage— especially because the food she makes is shy of sugar and flour and has those nifty Weight Watchers points accounted for. The backbone

---

63 "New Diet Winners," *Consumer Reports*, June 2007.

64 "You'll eat essentially the same food for breakfast, lunch, and snacks, and change up options for dinner. By decreasing the variety of food eaten throughout the day, you'll decrease the chance for the hedonistic rampages that can be so dangerous." Michael Roizen and Mehmet Oz, *You: On a Diet* (New York: Free Press, 2006), 237.

65 Breakfast can be 1 cup cooked rice; ½ cup (before cooking) oatmeal, kasha, or other hot multigrain cereal; or six ounces of potato. Lunch is almost always 2 cups salad and 1 tablespoon oil. All three meals include four ounces of protein.

66 Overnight Oatmeal: In slow cooker, combine 8 cups water, 2 cups steel-cut oats, ⅓ cup each dried cranberries and chopped apricots, and salt to taste. Cook on low 7 to 8 hours until oats are tender and creamy. Makes 8 1-cup servings, 4 Weight Watchers points each. To reheat, add a little water or milk and heat in microwave.

of her week's menus falls back on certain dishes: black bean and corn salad, edamame bean salad, applesauce, pudding/yogurt, her famous sweet potato and apple casserole, and ground-turkey spaghetti sauce.

Weight Watchers wasn't always that way. Mimi's first experience, over thirty years ago, had no variation in the meals participants were required to fix for themselves. "I asked for a Weight Watchers membership as my college graduation present. I followed it religiously for a year. That was in the days when you had to eat liver once a week, but I did it. I lost seventy-five pounds."

It was Mimi's first and last experience of shopping in the misses' sections.

Wendy reposted her profile on Match.com, Yahoo!, and Craigslist, and heard from a string of men who made her snicker even as they pissed her off. One man wrote that he was sixty-five years "young." Another asked her to go on a ten-mile bike ride—but his profile stated that he weighed 130 pounds and didn't want to date a woman who weighed more than 140 pounds. She had specified her age requirements as being within five years of her forty-seven and put up several recent photos of herself, clearly weighing far more than 140 pounds. Were these guys mass emailing every new posting without looking at profiles? Such indiscriminate responses stripped her of all the specialness—her sense of humor, her wide cultural interests, her willingness to take on new challenges like swimming and jewelry-making, her red hair, green eyes, and great smile—that she had carefully crafted in her profiles.

Mimi and I began getting twice-a-day phone calls on weekends from Wendy, who assumed we'd be home. It made me curse cell phones. They're scalpels to someone who likes silence, and most weekends I was boarding a dog and writing. Mimi, Katie, and I disliked Saturday night as much as any single woman, but we were more catholic in our unhappiness. We wished we had a best girlfriend who lived nearby to go to the movies with or that we were more motivated to go to the movies alone; we were stressed and tired from our weeks, which added to the lack of motivation; we enjoyed most of our weekend until Saturday night crept up on us, a purgatory we had pretty much forgotten in the intervening seven days. I disliked them because I was so often in prison with a second dog that was suffering homesickness. Prison is not good for my eating. I start to feel like I deserve instant gratification because there's no other gratification I can get away for. For me, food *is* instant gratification.

And yes, too often we have felt we deserve something for being alone. And too often we've gone grocery shopping and brought home either legal-but-lethal or criminal[67] food. But we didn't take our Saturday nights alone as personal failures. "I hate not being very important to someone," Wendy told me when I congratulated her on a second half-hour visit to the gym at seven thirty on a frosty November Saturday night. "I know I'm not unimportant, and it's just a night out of the weekend. But . . ." She sighed heavily. "Not a word from the Invisible Man. I don't get why he wants to go to this Thanksgiving thing. He says I should be dating other guys, that he's too busy to call me, so what's the point? Is he that desperate for a meal?"

"I dunno, honey. I'm not in a place right now where I can deal with men. You've been hurt twice, badly, in the last year. You might feel better if you didn't date for a while."

Lindsay, Mimi, and I kept making the point that until she was comfortable enough to make herself happy, she wasn't going to "find"

---

67 Legal-but-lethal food is that which is on the edge of one's food plan and should not be allowed in the house. Katie has to guard against cheese, bananas, and deli meats; Mimi can't have chocolate, peanut butter, or raisin bread in the house, and sticks either to Weight Watchers, Skinny Cows, or melting half the carton of low-fat ice cream in the sink. Lindsay targets anything made by Nabisco and Frito-Lay as legal-but-lethal, and Wendy's list includes, among other items, tortilla chips (with salsa and cheese, she calls this the "trifecta of delight"), pizza, and cheese. It's rare that I eat one serving of peanuts, peanut butter, or Grape-Nuts.

happiness in a man. Wendy knew this—intellectually. Then the cycle would start over. For her, Thanksgiving brought the threat of candles glowing in every Williamsburg window, fairy lights on High Street, and miles of pine boughs and red velvet ribbons.

"It sucks to live in a place that's famous for Christmas," she complained. "You can't leave the house without seeing couples, couples, couples. Parties, parties, parties."

"I live in New York," I said. "I know what it's like, believe me. At six o'clock at night, it seems like everyone is dressed up in black velvet party dresses and high heels and furs, stepping into town cars. I'm schlepping back from the last dog of the day in sweatpants and a camouflage flap hat and haven't showered in two days. It's a hard time. You just have to make *your* night to dress up and be one of the lucky people. It doesn't have to be for a guy, you know."

"I know. But when I was a kid, and even now, I feel more rejected at Christmas. I always identified with *A Charlie Brown Christmas*: 'I know nobody likes me. Why do we have to have a holiday season to emphasize it?'"

I wasn't surprised to read in her blog the next day that she ordered a pizza. "It was low fat," she wrote. Mimi called me on Sunday night to tell me the upshot of my attempt to assure Wendy she could find or invent an occasion befitting Williamsburg's glories. "She said it was a tiny pizza. Smaller than a dinner plate and no more than 660 calories. Then she felt sick afterwards."

"Ah," I said. "The old 'It was good to be reminded of that feeling' justification. Right up there with 'I got the craving out of my system.'"

"And 'I threw the last part away,'" she added.

"Along with 'I'll skip breakfast tomorrow.'"

"Don't forget 'At least it's out of the house.'" We snickered and went on to discuss the annual what-do-I-get-my-parents-for-Christmas dilemma.

Sometimes the best way to pull out of a food tailspin is to get a new bee in our bonnets, one we feel we have more control over and that will distract us from the desire to eat. Wendy is a champion at that.

Don't get me wrong: any one of us could be be obsessing over one thing or another at any moment. The difference is that we get through manias—Katie devotes herself to the latest television show or social networking website like a compass stuck at true north, Mimi replants her tiny herb garden according to each full-moon candle spell, I had an eBay quest at least every other month, Lindsay checks job listings at the Association of Higher Education several times a day. A mania lasts a week or a month and then it's over. You can, with effort, limit it, the way Mimi and I played too many dumb computer games when we didn't want to think—one of the addict's best options to avoid using her drug of choice. Obsession, on the other hand, is static, a constant and clawing state of mind, another symptom of holes in the psyche. Obsessions and manias are invaluable signs of where and how incomplete is the ego.

Wendy shopped. Each change in her body was a reason to get more, stretching her finances another centimeter they could barely accomodate. Every other post she wrote for her blog discussed trying to deal with the bins and piles of clothes in what could have been her dining room. She was a Goldilocks who couldn't decide what fit.

We all go through the clothing thing. Mimi kept a few beloved smaller sizes, and Katie purged hers. I kept my smaller sizes, classic clothes that wouldn't go out of fashion, and I'd be goddammed if I gave up on fitting into them. We packed this stuff up and got it out of our way whereas Wendy tortured herself with the mess.

It could have been genetic. Wendy's parents kept a stuffed baby fawn in the closet. "When I mention it's a bit odd, my mom says, 'Why is that odd? We keep it there because of the cat.' The cat has been dead for five years."

Wendy *suffered* from her clashing desires to get more and get rid of. She was convinced that one of the reasons Cal and Mark broke up with her was because of her clutter. It seemed her drives always came back to her pursuit of weight loss (the calorie-counting and points, the cups and halves, the clothes, the gym, the scale, the photos, the blogging, the new makeup, the new hair cut), and her weight loss always came back to men.

Each particular of weight loss became so obsessional that it partly obscured (to herself, at any rate) the obsession to find a man. "My scale has ranged from 263 to 255 in the past thirty-six hours. I'd just like it to be a certain number. Before I left for Weight Watchers, my scale said 257. The Weight Watchers scales said 258.8." Wendy also had several gym scales to consult and not infrequent visits to her doctors, making her weight notoriously complicated.

So was her food. Wendy's participation in Weight Watchers was mostly, in her Goldilocks world, to batten down a single, final, authoritative weight. After she weighed in, she had a ritual that, of course, involved Five Continents. "I selected the biggest pieces of huevos rancheros with the biggest piece of cheese on it," she blogged on a mid-November Saturday. I was faint with lust reading it: the last leaves in Brooklyn were bristling in a stiff wind that portended winter, and I was longing for something warming and fatty. "It was really delicious but I wanted more. I went back and got my fruits and vegetables and strolled past the breakfast bar again. I got two more pieces to go. AND I picked up four double chocolate cookies that they sell by the package, the smallest one at $2.04." Then she went back to the meeting for discussions of point-wise recipes and not going grocery shopping on an empty stomach.

Her blog reports of eating out were Gordian knots of points: "We split a pork carnita dinner (all meat), refried beans (with an extra order), lettuce, guacamole (about a 1/4 c. total) and I probably had about ten to twelve chips" or "I did have ¼ of a slice of pound cake today but I've been bringing in an apple and a banana each day along with a controlled lunch."

"Am I more attractive and lovable losing weight?" Wendy asked. It's an interesting and universal question in the dating world. Even the thinnest man or woman might wonder if he'd gain from shaving off his mustache or having a second piercing in her ear. To question if a pound or two can make one more attractive is not that unreasonable in how it affects confidence. And the answer to Wendy is yes, but not as much as women think. "Why wouldn't I want to go away with you for Thanksgiving?" Mark said when he finally called and she pushed him on why he'd broken up with her but still wanted to see her. "You're great company. I love being with you."

To someone like Wendy, whose flailing for self-improvement was caused by her drive to get a boyfriend or was an escape from not having one, that "love" was as confusing as parking signs in New York City. I was going through the same confusion with Scott and not unlike my breakups with him three and four years earlier, Wendy was hitting the Internet in a hard, lost-girl fashion. I was baffled how to respond to the email she sent to the Angry Fat Girlz bloggers.

> I'm thinking of putting up a new personal ad. I'm supposedly going to have some new photos from a professional photographer. What qualities would you write about me? Remember, we're dealing with men who are not known so we have to think like them a bit. I'm notoriously bad about writing about myself and when I look at the other women's profiles, I think, "they seem fun and have a life" and I feel very dull in comparison. Also, any suggestions for describing my body?

Uh, I kept thinking as the message waited for an answer, *you could be fun, you could have a life.* "Deep down inside," she had blogged earlier, "all of us want to be accepted and it hurts to know that our weight keeps people away from us. We'd all like to think we are more than our weight," and yet here she was, putting herself up for sale without knowing what her "more" was or how to gloss over the ninety pounds she had yet to lose in addition to the hundred she'd been victorious in shedding. Why not take a full body shot and not worry about describing your body?

My brain wheeled with the things I could have said, but in the end I advised her to post what *she* wanted from a man. Maybe— possibly—such a list would have landed her a man she wouldn't have to twist herself into a different person for, that she wouldn't have had to time-share with kids, work, or another woman.

On the Sunday before Thanksgiving, the morning after seeing *Marie Antoinette* and going out for Mexican food with Mark on a "just friends" date, and four days before they were going to Pulaski, Wendy threw gasoline on the fire.

She hadn't heard from Cal since May or June, when he quit agonizing over missing Wendy and apologizing for staying with the woman Wendy called the "she-male." But now he was calling her again. When she grabbed the phone, she saw his number on the LCD and for two rings considered whether she ought to answer. She was curious about what he would say and felt she had nothing to lose. She would salve some of her hurt and loneliness by calling him a bastard and hanging up on him.

All it took was "I wanted to wish you a happy Thanksgiving, Wen. I've been thinking about the party at your cousin's and the Comfort Inn in Pulaski." She invited him over, to which he answered he was in her parking lot, and in what seemed like fifteen seconds, she was on top of him, fucking both their brains out until she stopped and said, huskily, "Tell me I'm better than her. Tell me I'm sexier and better in bed."

What was he gonna say, as close to orgasm as he was?

Mimi was impressed with the way her Weight Watchers leader had set up the room, with paper plates at each seat of the conference table and a card table with bowls and plates labeled "mashed potatoes," "turkey," "cranberry sauce," "pumpkin pie," each filled with different-sized pieces of paper. The leader had them go through the buffet line and choose what they would select for Thanksgiving dinner, then went over the points for the portion each person selected and showed them the size they should be aiming for of the food they'd be served.

"Go ahead and have pie," she said, "but keep it to a one-and-a-half-inch slice and don't put whipped cream on it. If you make great dressing, think about skipping the potatoes, or vice versa. Remember this is a holiday not a pig-out. Try to keep your mind on the company."

Mimi found the portion sizes fascinating and resolved to skip gravy, mashed potatoes, rolls, and cranberries. She would make her casserole, and she loved the cornbread stuffing and pecan pie her hostess and sister Wiccan, Jolene, always served. Mimi would save her points for them.

I went to my potluck with my pie and a ton of Brussels sprouts. There was no plum pudding or mincemeat pie left when I went home.

Katie and I didn't get pumpkin pie at our celebrations, but the stores were still open and Entenmann's did in a pinch.

Jalen and Lindsay got to her parents' house too early. Like a good son-in-law, he settled in to watch a football game, and she joined her mom and sisters in the fragrant kitchen. Janice was wearing skinny black jeans and Alison a short denim skirt with cabled tights. *At least we're all in bulky sweaters*, Lindsay thought, but as the big pot for potatoes added plumes of steam to the heat of the oven and Crock-Pot, she knew the sweaters would be coming off.

"You look goood," Alison cooed. "You've lost more weight." Alison lived in Minneapolis, and they hadn't seen each other since the wedding.

"Thanks," Lindsay said. "You look good, too." She had prepared this response in order not to fall to her knees in floods of questions at each compliment. *Do you really, really think so? Can you see it in my butt? How about my thighs?*

Their mom walked by with a relish tray. "I've already had a couple of carrots," she said. "I was starving. Do you think the men would like some snacks, too?"

Janice took the tray, the bride eager to join her groom, and seeing nothing to do in the kitchen, Lindsay followed. Janny was perched on Evan's lap as the Lions got a third down. The men hadn't been going hungry before the arrival of the celery and olives. Mom had set out onion dip and potato chips, salsa and Tostitos. And a floral china plate, Lindsay saw with glee, of snowman and jack-o'-lantern Peeps.

Jack-o'-lanterns! They'd be just a tiny bit stale, just the way, as everyone in the family knew, she liked them. Ripened to perfection.

The naked trees on the mountains driving into Pulaski always give Wendy the willies. Their famished arms seemed to try to snatch her back, reminding her of the couple of generations of Wickses buried in Pulaski's and nearby Hillsville's cemeteries: two dead of black lung, a suicide, a blast furnace victim. The stories of her paternal grandfather are of a harsh, brutal man, but at least he got his family out of the mines and foundries. As an itinerate market farmer, he was poorer than his brothers, and when her dad was growing up, the family never had a place they called home for long, but they all had an up-and-out bent bred into their natures for which she had to be grateful.

"They call me Deesie," she warned Mark as they drove into town. "Actually, my mother calls me Dee-Rett. She believes everyone should be called by versions of both names. Wendy Harriet—Dee-Rett. But everyone else calls me Deesie."

"Okay, Deesie. Anything else you want me to know?"

"Yeah. *You* don't call me Deesie. Elsewise I'll tell my mom your full name."

"Wait!" Mark Luke John Nixon grabbed her arm. "We gotta look at the VFW. It's a classic."

"You'll see a lot of those false-front places heresabout," she said.

"We can drive 'round in the morning if you want. Go up and see where the Boss Men lived."

"'Heresabout'?"

"Ah'm goin' ta see mah people, son. Ah'm goin' ta Cousin Tanny's, where mah aunt Darla'll make jokes about us bein' salt 'n' pepper, Darla and Dessie. Get it?" She slapped him on the thigh and pulled up to a white and stone tract house distinguishable from its neighbors for the wishing well on the front lawn. The driveway was populated by three motorcycles and a flat-bottomed fishing boat on a trailer.

Mark was absorbed into the crowd like water into a sponge, carried off by Tanny to meet Wendy's mother. This meant she was left to the clutches of her aunt and uncle, Darla and Floyd. "Oh. Mah. Gawd!" Aunt Darla yelled. "You all come look at Dee-Rett! She's thin!"

Aunt Darla pronounced "thin" as two syllables.

"What *haaave* you been doing to yourself, child?"

"I just lost some weight, Aunt Dar. Just thirty pounds or so since I saw you in July."

"An' all dressed up and with a new friend, too," she said knowingly.

"Well . . . I have to admit I've fallen in love with Talbots."

"Ah can *see* that! Ah *love* that jacket." She fingered the lapel of Wendy's navy blue blazer. "What size is it, honey?"

Wendy was exhausted. There were twenty or thirty people at this party and she'd only survived two of them.

"I don't right remember. The label might have been torn off. I got it for twelve dollars. Could you excuse me? It's been a long drive, and I need to use the bathroom."

Wendy locked the door and slumped against it. She was perspiring, and her hair was matted along her hairline, her blazer wrinkled in the back from being in the car. She needed to pee, she needed a Diet Coke, and she needed to see if Cal had called her back. She smiled when she saw his number on her cell phone.

"You interested in NASCAR?" Uncle Floyd was asking Mark.

"We have races up here over the summer. You and Deesie'd be more than welcome."

"I've never been a fan," Mark said, "but I'd like to check out the fishing."

A chorus of ah's went up. Mark was in. He was on his own.

"So how are you really?" Tanny asked Wendy. Wendy turned, and Tanny could see her eyes were red from crying. "Uh-oh."

"Why are men such idiots?" Wendy asked.

"Did you and Mark have a fight?"

"No. No. We're past fighting. We're just friends. I'm in love with somebody else. I always have been."

"And he's not—?"

"In love with me? Yeah, he is. I think. He said so. That's what makes it hard. But he's living with this witch, this . . . this . . . *vampire.* 'Carol,' " she said in a baby voice and with a toss of her head. "*Carol* does her best not to let him out of her sight, but she doesn't always do a very good job." She started to cry then. Tanny took her in her arms and petted her hair.

"It sounds awful, honey. Awful."

"Yeah," Wendy whispered. "Sometimes he slips up. Like saving his cell phone messages."

"Deesie, don't you think—"

"Ah *think*," she cut in, all those Wickses stretching in their graves at Dora Cemetery and thickening her accent to the viscosity of Aunt Dar's candied yams, "ah'm gonna pay 'em *both* back. Ah'll get thin, you wait. Then he'll regret it. And *her* . . . Ah might let her know a thing or two about Cal."

She took a long sniff and pulled away from Tanny. "Is there gonna be salad today?"

NINE

December

The Body's Politics

L osing weight in order to get a man never works," Mimi said as we fingered filigree earrings at a Union Square Holiday Market kiosk. We had met a half hour earlier at Penn Station, for the first time. It was my fiftieth birthday. I wanted to share it with someone who had crossed this boundary, two old maids who had blogged their way into being bubulas. We had gotten an email the night before about Wendy's new war on men, and between cooing over Christmas ornaments and jewelry, we relished the latest pronouncement. "You either give up halfway through or gain it all back," Mimi said as we walked on to a display of Polish handblown ornaments.

If anyone would know, I learned that day, it's Mimi.

Fine-boned and clear-skinned as a Dresden doll, Mimi is the prettiest of the Angry Fat Girls. She is also the daintiest. At five feet three inches tall, she has spent much of her life not only shopping for large sizes but petite ones as well. Her choices have gotten more numerous over the years but dressing room mirrors send her into spirals.

Larger sizes were just beginning to claim a share of the fashion market in 1980, when Mimi moved to Chapel Hill, North Carolina, to work in the Health Sciences Library at the university. She lived in a parlor-floor apartment, her first one-bedroom in this, her second post-graduate school job. It was a peeling Victorian on a quiet street off Mount Carmel Church Road, a name she came to view as prescient for Elijah's warning on that ancient ground: "...if the Lord be God, follow him: but if Baal, then follow him." She loved her apartment's hardwood floors, the bay window in what had been the parlor, the scuffed oak table she had found in Carrboro and sanded and painted herself, and the closets that were big enough to fit several of her 245-pound selves into.

In many ways, her seven years in Chapel Hill should have been among the best of her life. The winters were mild and the landscape was beautiful. In accepting the job, she'd accepted a promotion and had been promoted since. The choirmaster at her Episcopalian church took a great sigh and turned his eyes heavenward when she auditioned. "Thank God," Stephen said. "Our alto section has been saved."

She became active in St. Alban's, not only in the choir but in its spiritual outreach, going on and later helping to organize retreats. St. Alban's provided a pool of like-minded women she found herself, for the first and last time in her life, doing things with—shopping, going to recitals and concerts in Durham, exploring Raleigh, and having brunch after Sunday services. Professionally and socially, Mimi felt she belonged.

She hated every minute of her life.

It's not easy being more than a hundred pounds overweight when you're surrounded by medical school professors and students. She saw every article on obesity in every periodical the library subscribed to, and she saw the looks when she went to the cafeteria.

She had arrived at the University of North Carolina two years earlier weighing 160 pounds, fifteen pounds more than her lowest adult weight, achieved through Weight Watchers in graduate school.

In her first two years in Chapel Hill, she gained eighty-five pounds. The shame felt like another fifty pounds on her aching body.

She entered a rigorous weight-loss program at Dicken-Harriman Hospital. Six weeks of behavioral therapy followed by three twelve-week sessions of supervised fasting with six-week breaks between each fast. She lost a hundred pounds and her hair in ten months, developed acute gastritis, and despite classes in transition taught by a nutritionist, gained her weight back within a year.

Her misery was so potent that people started to notice. "Is everything alright at work?" Mary Jo, one of the priests' wives asked. "How was your trip home? Are your parents well?"

"I *hate* myself," Mimi blurted. She was shocked that she's said it out loud, said it to another person. "My mother couldn't *believe* how much weight I'd gained. It was the most humiliating conversation I've had with her since I lived at home. I wanted to die." She stopped and considered whether to say it all. "Sometimes," she said slowly, "I stand in front of my mirror and think about how I'd do it. I'd slit my wrists, I think—or the dorsalis pedis artery." She smiled wryly. "Being a medical librarian hasn't helped me lose weight, but it's great for plotting suicide."

"Have you talked to anyone about this?" Mary Jo asked.

"Yeah. You."

"You need to talk to someone professional," she said. "You can't harbor self-hatred and suicidal thoughts."

Mimi knew about talk therapy, of course. Who didn't? But she had no idea how to march out and find the right person to talk to. No one she knew well had been in therapy, and her parents spoke of it as a scam. If you have a problem, she'd been taught, you take it to God.

"Maybe I should talk to someone at the church," Mimi answered. "The doctors can't help, and I can't help myself even to go back to Weight Watchers."

"Why don't you talk to Michael?" Mary Jo said. "I know I'm his wife, but everyone says he's a wonderful counselor. And . . . he's been worried about you, too. I know he'll want to help."

Mimi went into pastoral counseling with Michael Clark, going over her history of eating and how it had eroded her self-esteem. She told him how she had scared herself when she had dieted down to 145 pounds at the age of twenty-five.

"Everyone was going into the next stage of their life," she told him. "They'd already gone through the rights of passage—dating, breakups, living together. I was always buying engagement or wedding presents, and I'd never been on a date."

In the course of the next two years, they talked a lot about how she felt toward men. Was her eating a substitute for love? What if it wasn't about loving the taste and texture and temperature that filled her with a sense of connection to all of time? Could food and fat be the wall she put up to keep men away?

She didn't know. She'd had sex once, with a bus driver she met on a trip to Spain the summer she was at her thinnest. "It was painful," she said when Father Mike asked about it. "I bled profusely." He was sympathetic. That was the first session he ended with a hug and a recommendation that she read a book called *Becoming Orgasmic*.

Despite the obesity center's prohibition against doing a second round of fasts, Mimi entered the Dicken-Harriman program for a second time. She got through one twelve-week session and lost twenty-five pounds but had to quit because of chronic stomach cramps and constipation. Instead, she joined the hospital's WiseWeight group and counted calories and fats, minutes on a stationary bike, and ounces of water. Slowly, she lost more weight. She liked being able to occasionally find clothes in the petite sections, liked her increasing energy. She took a trip to Scotland with her mother, and enjoyed walking in the mountains and cobbled-street towns.

Father Mike kept recommending books. *Everything You Always Wanted to Know About Sex and Were Afraid to Ask*, *The Art of Sensual Loving*—even, oddly, Gael Greene's *Delicious Sex*. "Appetite is natural," he assured her. "Let's see what happens to your cravings for chocolate as you fulfill another appetite."

Sometimes he dropped by her apartment with a novel he thought she'd enjoy or a CD of choral works. He would stay for iced tea, and they'd talk about the choir or a parishioner's illness she'd investigated for him. One dank July evening in 1984, he dropped in with a bottle of Liebfraumilch and a video cassette. "I think you'll like this," he said, handing her the sturdy ceramic bottle and the black rental box. "I know you like sweet things, and this movie reminds me a lot of you."

She poured the wine and took out the cassette. *The Devil in Miss Jones.*

She did not find it impressive and asked, rather crankily, why all the naughty stuff featured heroines named Justine?

Father Mike didn't answer and didn't seem to notice when she got up to wash their wineglasses during the last sex scene. She returned in time to see Georgina Spelvin pleading with her milquetoast, fly-obsessed roommate in hell.

"Some people might think I stepped over a line," he said, "but I wanted you to see what pleasure is like, what a man can teach a woman." He slipped the video back into its case. "Think about it, Mimi. Think of all the possibilities that await you as you lose more weight."

His tongue tasted of stale wine and, faintly, toothpaste. It wasn't unpleasant, but it was deeply disturbing. She wondered what it would be like to do that with his hand under her shirt.

It was her thirty-fifth birthday and she weighed 211 pounds.

Her involvement with Michael Clark—which consisted of making out on an irregular basis—continued for the next two years. It was hell: a relationship that could not speak its own name. She and Mary Jo were friends. Trying to act natural with her was a struggle. Those were the days before the Internet and free long-distance calling, so she couldn't talk to old friends and she certainly couldn't confide in friends at church. The only good thing, besides how thrilling it was to be held and kissed, was that she maintained her 211 pounds.

"Now you know why I took a day off from work to spend your birthday with you." She laughed dryly. "I'll do anything I can to help birthday haters like their birthday."

On another languidly hot day, waiting for thunderstorms to roll in, Mike invited Mimi to his house. They sat on his porch and drank sweet tea. "There's something I have to tell you," he finally said. "While Mary Jo and Amanda have been visiting her parents, I've moved all my stuff into an apartment. She's getting home in a couple of hours. I'll tell her tonight."

Mimi was silent. Hope and guilt and grief were doing a square dance in her chest. Mary Jo would be devastated and so would Amanda, a chubby fourteen-year-old Mimi adored. And yet—to go away to the mountains with Michael or to a concert—to make dinner for him . . .

"I wanted you to be the first to know," he went on. "Mary Jo and Amanda are going to need you."

Their need, which was great, was the end of her involvement with Father Clark. He dropped by once or twice and then disappeared from her life. She quit the choir at St. Alban's and stopped attending services. Her weight rocketed. In the summer of 1987, she took a job in Burlington, Vermont. It was a step up professionally, but in that lonely, confused winter, with more snow than she'd ever imagined possible, she spent nights and weekends stewing in blame for being a two-faced, lying adulteress.

From the time the maples turned to the time the lilacs were in bloom, Mimi gained ninety pounds.

The story of Father Mike carried us through a search for a dumpling place I couldn't find and a terrible Chinese dive lunch and back up Mott to Mulberry, where I had my heart set on sugar. "Men are sooo not a motivation for losing weight," she concluded as we nibbled at desserts—hazelnut gelato for her, Italian ricotta cheesecake for me—in Ferrara's. "I don't think Wendy's ever going to get that."

I stood in front of the pastry case and said, "Do I look really fat?"

My reflection in the gold-veined mirror along the opposite wall looked like a portly clown.

Mimi sighed. Now it was Wendy *and* Frances who were annoying her.

"You look good," she said.

"It's the trousers, isn't it? They're too big."

"They are too big, yes." At that, she lifted her camera and took a picture of me. I was smiling the secret smile of someone who has undergrown her current favorite item of clothing. I was also ashamed of putting her through that vampirish series of questions about size. The question "Do I look fat?" is a lie because what we really want to know is "Do I look thin?" followed by an infinitude of adjectives that we rarely give voice to. Am I pretty? Am I smart? Am I good at my job? Am I nice? Am I lovable? Just *how* much am I these things? The answer "no" to the question of size is not truly reassuring because we forced it out of our acquaintance. Would Mimi have had the brute honesty to say yes to one of her favorite authors whom she had just met for the first time in order to celebrate her friend's fiftieth birthday?

Perhaps only Lindsay would have cut me off or answered yes. She was the least tolerant of us and had learned not to indulge the games played by people she loved.

As overweight as I was on my birthday, I'm six inches taller than Mimi, and my bones are so strong that my bone density is literally off the chart. I also walked dogs for a living and lived in a city where picking up a prescription or getting a quart of milk adds another half mile of walking a day. My questions about my size were deeply insensitive to a woman who is so short and so broad, in so much pain from her knee that much of the world beyond cars and trains is grievously inaccessible to her. Mimi goes to business conventions and Wiccan events that are important to her and to see her parents in Florida, but she has to brace herself for the humiliation and discomfort of airplanes and passengers alike. With a trip to Florida coming up in ten days, she was hoping against probability for the magic empty middle seat.

Some months later, in April 2007, Mimi mentioned in an email that she was too furious to think about some other matter. She was reading an MSNBC message board discussion of a recent article on etiquette and planning for the fat air traveler. The snarkiness of the responses was a flashback to her most recent flight, of bambling down the aisle to her seat, trying not to look at the two businessmen in A and B. I emailed back that she *must* stop reading the message board, then took a look at it for myself. The article was balanced, but it was the ensuing remarks that had Mimi shaking and crying, she admitted in the next email. Almost seven hundred posts had turned up and a fair share of them reflected thin smugness for the out-of-control fatty: "Put down the fork, get your duff off the couch and start moving . . . and exercise a little discipline too," read one, and the responders went on to meaner polemics: "Not only are our airline seats being taken over by ripples of pudge, but our tax dollars are going to be spent on the healthcare for people that just can't put down the butterfinger [sic]."

Then we had one of the most draining conversations I've had about living in big bodies.

"So why am I still fat?" Mimi asked before saying good-bye. "I don't get it. We are despised and it's not like I didn't know it. Why would anyone choose to be hated?"

Indeed, obese people, and particularly women, are increasingly at risk of becoming Public Enemy Number One. In 1997, former surgeon general C. Everett Koop urged that ". . . this war on obesity must continue unabated."[68] At the 2003 Obesity Summit, U.S. surgeon general Richard Carmona proclaimed that childhood obesity ". . . is every bit as threatening to us as is the terrorist threat we face today."[69]

---

68   His statement was made as spokesman for Shape Up America! in response to the news that Wyeth-Ayerst Laboratories was taking Phen-fen off the market.

69   Radley Balko, "The Terror of Fat," *National Post*, June 16, 2004.

Some two-thirds of our fellow Americans consider our fat to be indicative of lack of self-control, laziness, moral deviance, self-indulgence, and incorrigibility,[70] while comedians and phobic bloggers have no compunction about telling jokes and calling us names. Any formerly fat person has listened to thin people whisper about why Maura isn't being promoted or what a shame Chris has let herself go. Most people's defense is to live in a carefully guarded zone of silence. But it takes little more than a random link on the Yahoo! home page to have the troops from the war on obesity pour into that most tender and fraught of all personal vulnerabilities.

There are, however, others who do not live behind silence in order to avoid another skirmish. The article that caused Mimi's mini-breakdown, Harriet Baskas's "Squeezed to Meet You,"[71] closely follows the tips that the National Association to Advance Fat Acceptance gives for airplane travel: book off-peak hour flights, buy two tickets, fly first class or reserve aisle or window seats, and tell the airline in advance that, if possible, you'd like to be next to an empty seat.[72] Baskas goes one better than NAAFA, advising large travelers to be friendly to airline personnel and their neighbors. "You might end up shedding some stereotypes as well."

Mimi was just back from New Orleans, an amulet of sea salt, mugwort, and allspice under her shirt to attract the empty middle seat. Each March, Mimi works with other solitary Wicca practitioners to prepare for the vernal equinox sabbat of Ostara, the goddess of the dawn and

---

70   J. Eric Oliver, *Fat Politics: The Real Story Behind America's Obesity Epidemic* (New York: Oxford University Press, 2006), 74.

71   http://www.msnbc.msn.com (accessed April 2, 2007).

72   As of April 15, 2009, United Airlines has taken NAAFTA and the MSNBC etiquette points literally. A passenger who cannot fit in a single seat, fasten the seat belt with a single extender, and/or put the armrest down, will be forced to purchase an extra seat or upgrade if s/he cannot be reaccommodated next to an empty seat. http://www.united.com/page/article/0,6722,52985,00.html.

of spring, married at the feast to the sun god. On the night of the Sap Moon, Mimi, in her alter ego as Asterië, and five other women and two men cast a circle in the backyard of her friend Helen's farmhouse an hour outside of the city, invoking Callisto, a woman changed into a bear, Ursa Major, because of various sexual transgressions in the stories told about her. They turned their faces to the stars and traced the constellation of Virgo, associated with Persephone, whose reemergence from the underworld brings spring to the earth.

March in Louisiana meant Helen's—or Selene, in the Circle—overgrown yard was abundant with magick from the flowers Philadelphia wouldn't see for another month or see at all. Azaleas and magnolias, hibiscus, passion flowers, camellias, ginger, and the all-important thorn apple, one of the three witches' weeds along with mandrake and henbane, vied for primacy in the night. As High Priestess, Selene burned the dried petals of the cornflower and alder twigs, and the circle dipped their hands three times in a basin of water dancing with dandelion leaves and petals, purifying themselves before the four compass points and the virgin stars.

Selene chanted a prayer of thanks for the lengthening days and warming soil, and called upon the offerings placed on the altar to honor creativity, protection, tranquillity, and prosperity—a knot of parsley, the eggs she and Mimi had dyed in vegetables the day before, a bouquet of narcissus and vervain. The men drummed to the Sap Moon and Mimi/Asterië, moved by the rhythms and the occasional call of the mockingbird, found herself dancing, naked, arms outstretched to embrace the bear in the sky. Her knees didn't bother her and her friends, intoxicated by this inspired abandon, began to sing, tunelessly, their histories and dedications within the art of white magick. Mimi weighed 268 pounds, eight more than she had in June, six months earlier, when we initiated Angry Fat Girlz.

And yet, amid the sky-clad group growing ever closer to her offering of white-white skin, full-nippled heavy breasts, and swinging belly, their hands touching her for the connection she radiated with Terpsichore, she had never felt more comfortable in her own skin. This was the core truth of Mimi. She had a genius for being absorbed in worship and a calling to be one priestess among many. This truth was light-years beyond the facts of the 140-pound twenty-four-year-old wearing her first business suit from Lord & Taylor, the woman who tries so hard to appreciate the feel and look of a fuzzy pink sweater, the woman who runs a prestigious medical library's website. For a glorious, unself-conscious twenty minutes, she was Asterië rather than the woman who steps on a scale once a week to stare at a different kind of truth.

But she did not get an empty middle seat on the trip home. Her back and neck, despite ritual, despite parsley and mugwort, ached for a week after.

Mimi describes herself as being thoughtful, creative, and smart, and it showed in her writing and blog page layouts, her interest in web design, and her work as an herbalist and candle maker. She's the AFG who calls to listen when one of us is in a tough patch, and we lean on her. On the other hand, she lists the "worst things about [her]self" as being self-critical, lazy, and fat.

Can one's *self* be fat? As defined by the Encarta Dictionary, no, not really. It defines self as "somebody's personality or an aspect of it, especially as perceived by others." Or do others see our fat and ladle on the associated faults until we forget that fat is a physical adjective, applicable to clouds and bodies alike? Is fat shorthand for a long list of things we don't like or have come to believe?

I brought this up with Lindsay one morning. "It's the 'I *am*' that gets me," I said as I pulled on heavy socks. The weird weather had turned frigid, and dressing had turned into a long ordeal. "I am funny. I am smart. I am talented . . ." I trickled off. It sounded dumb to sit there telling myself I'm good with dogs or a good cook.

"I know what you mean. It sounds so . . . self-justifying."

"Yeah," I said, "and, like, you're saying it in advance of someone denying it, and then if they do, like, say, 'You're not smart. Gore Vidal is smart,' then you have to take that affirmation off your list."

"*Am*," Lindsay reminded me, is a weak verb. "That's the second week of freshman comp."

"I think I like the verb *have* better,'" I said. "'I have intelligence. I have talent.' Even I have fat.'"

"It's like your best qualities are on reserve at the bank," Lindsay answered. "Like, you might not be able to write today, but you have talent to draw on tomorrow."

"Yes!" I said, stamping my feet into my snow boots. "*Am* is subject to opinion. *Have* is more personal, more of a claim to your self. 'I have fat . . . but I also have a nun doll collection. I have fat . . . but I have a plan to get rid of it.'"

"To have" is to say this or that is mine, I thought as I leashed Daisy and headed out into the windchill. It's a word of responsibility and specificity. "I am loving" is very different from "I have love." "I have love" can mean one has love to give or one has love coming in, like a hiker whose canteen might or might not be empty. You might have to extend the sentence to get it right, but in doing so, you are forced to consider the alternative: "I have love to give. I have love in my life," asks you to acknowledge the sources.

The words that go well with "I am" don't go well with "to have": funny, smart, generous, a good mother/daughter/aunt. You're forced to reword, and the rewording is a claim of reciprocity. To say "I have a daughter" is also to say that your daughter has a mother. If you're gunning for more specificity, "to have" forces you to act on it—use it, do it. "I have good parenting skills" provokes an assessment of whether you use them or not. "I have love for my daughter" asks if you've shown it lately.

"'To have' is a tool," I told Lindsay the next morning.

"Then 'to be' is multiple personality." She laughed. "It switches from being a good friend to being a good mother and back to smart."

She rang off because she was going into the library, leaving me to rumble this around some more.

"To have," I decided, is a marriage to one's self, that arsenal of merits and faults that makes us viable, liable, and human.

It could be about time to get down on my knees in front of a mirror and propose to myself.

If the second word in defining ourselves is *fat*, are we using it instead of lazy, gluttonousness, self-indulgent, dirty, smelly, out of control, diseased, stupid, voluminous, a drain on society? And if that's true, how could Mimi carry around 340 pounds on her tiny frame, serving on the board of the national medical librarians' association, earning promotions, tending a garden, putting together Ikea furniture (she was a whiz with a drill), traveling to Spain, Switzerland, Scotland?

It's *hard work* simply to live with fifty or 250 extra pounds. To do it and stand up to address one's peers or get out of bed and go to work for eight hours is anything but lazy, self-indulgent, stupid, out of control, or sick.

She was Atlas carrying the heavens, not on her shoulders but in her belly.

Only in its usage as part of the vocabulary of immunology does *self* refer to the body, how our corporeal selves recognize tissues and organs as their own.

Since Mimi's experiences with Michael Clark, she would regain weight when she approached 211 pounds. She's gotten down to 222, 220, 215, but she regained whenever 211 was in sight. It was a psychological threshold and the only time she crossed it was fifteen years later, in 2001, when she let another man she thought she could trust guide her. But when Mimi gained, she didn't stop when 211 was safely off the scale's radar. Was she "immune," in a metaphorical sense, to weight loss? Did her body not recognize itself when she lost fat?

Was Mimi one of the people who should stop torturing herself with points, weekly weigh-ins, and using Weight Watchers tips such as asking for ten french fries instead of the full order?

From the get-go, dieters have at best a 10 percent chance of maintaining weight loss. Fat women have to ask themselves why they put themselves through the tedium, stress, labor, and loss of liberty that a diet induces. Increasingly, the evidence is that, as long as we eat nutritiously and exercise regularly, only the severely obese will suffer weight-related health consequences.

What, then, would it take for Mimi—Katie, Lindsay, Wendy, or me—to live at peace, even lovingly, with our big bodies? There are a number of organizations for people who achieved such a truce, pre-eminently NAAFA and HAES (Health at Every Size).[73] Twelve-step parlance calls fat acceptance "Fat Serenity." I haven't found much evidence of serenity, and acceptance into the fat club has been elusive in my efforts to unlock the secret of the body truce.

The fat acceptance community is as shy as morning glories at midnight. Keeping in mind the vicious responses to "Squeezed to Meet You," I can understand their reluctance. But so antithetical is the notion of weight loss to fat acceptance proponents that it's as though I had said nothing besides "I'm losing weight" in my requests to discuss either NAAFA's work or individual women's journeys toward coming to love their fat bodies.

My words were matches thrown into deep wells of fossilized anger. "I won't talk to you," one woman told me straight out after she had given me her phone number. "You don't understand the feminist political aspects of my work. You're one of the enemy."

I was adhering to my food plan and losing weight, but I weighed 232 pounds that day. How can I *not* support many of the fat acceptance philosophies?

An editor at BellaOnline passed my interest in speaking with women living in fat acceptance to an online group called Don't Tell Me What Size I Must Be. The referral prompted more anger at my

---

73   HAES promotes "Natural diversity in body shape and size; [the] Ineffectiveness and dangers of dieting for weight loss; [the] Importance of relaxed eating in response to internal body cues; [the] Critical contribution of social, emotional and spiritual as well as physical factors to health and happiness." Jon Robison, PhD, MS, "Health At Every Size: Toward a New Paradigm of Weight and Health," Medscape General Medicine, http//www.medscape .com/viewarticle/506299_print (accessed July 12, 2005).

supposed duplicity. How, I was asked, could I accept myself as a fat person *and* diet? By sharing their stories with me, they risked endorsing my double standard. Didn't I know dieting doesn't work? Look what had happened to me and look at the blog—Angry Fat Girlz—I was associated with. And finally, how could I only devote one chapter to the question of whether to diet or not?

Obviously, I had not shared the entire outline of my book, so there was no way that they could know that the question of the viability of dieting runs throughout our five stories. And I had asked for information, not a club card or validation; beyond that, while the seed for this book was my failure, my failure was partial. I did not, as that vaunted 90 percent do, gain all of my weight back. Nor do I think my twelve-step program and food plan failed. *I* failed. When the crisis came, I had not grown out of my fat history enough to stand up for myself.

Maybe Mimi is right: we *can* have fat personalities.

Certainly, the public figures within the fat acceptance movement, authors and/or popular bloggers have defined themselves as fat. "Fat," Lara Frater writes breathlessly, is "not something abnormal that must be eliminated at all costs, but the very essence of who I am!"[74] As an author who has written the Baedeker's guide to the planet of fat girls, finding a social life in the fat acceptance movement and a husband among Fat Admirers,[75] it is possible to see why she claims her size as her identity. Lara was more forthcoming about the chimerical process from body hatred to body embracement. "You know how they say there's a thin person inside every fat person?" she said in a slightly raspy voice that has definite charm and sex appeal. "Well, there's a fat person living inside me, and that's all there is. It's a thing I had to take

74   Laura Frater, *Fat Chicks Rule!* (Brooklyn: Ig Press, 2005), 12.

75   "Fat admirers (FAs) get off on the thrill of being surrounded and engulfed by fat partners . . . NAAFA supports FAs, believing 'that a preference for a fat partner is as valid as any other preference based on physical characteristics . . .'" Ibid., 189.

upon myself, to accept. I am fat. That's not going to change, and that's who I am. When I was trying to lose weight, I hated my body and myself. I *had* to love my body."

I puzzled over this business of *being* for weeks. One evening, walking Daisy and her extroverted, eighty-pound pal, Henry, I remembered a sister-in-law telling me that when she met me, I was bouncing from one piece of furniture to another in the living room, singing "I am pretty/Oh so pretty/I am pretty and witty and—*fat!*" I was in seventh grade when I danced and chanted this ditty, and sixteen when she told me her memory of it. I cramped with compassion for that girl, four years younger than I then was, performing her absolutely true feelings in equal measures of gaiety and self-mockery.

I was surprised when I looked the lyrics up. It is not "I *am* pretty" but "I *feel* pretty." I was devoted to Broadway musicals but had turned one of my all-time favorites into self-definition.

As a 240-pound high schooler who felt condemned to living in a stasis of desperately wanting and being locked out of getting, I should have envied the kid leaping around in her plaid uniform. That kid may have undermined pretty and witty, but she hadn't lost possession of them.

Relapsers punish and ghettoize themselves more than those who don't or rarely diet, or those who have been in relapse a long time. It is a different way of being fat and not a kind one. My therapist forbid me to take the bags I'd bought binge food in the night before and pick up litter with them, my self-punishment that further degraded me but was nice for the street I live on. As B.J., a friend of mine who had regained a lot of weight in a few months, prepared for her engagement party, I asked her if she'd found a cute outfit.

"Fff't," she exhaled. "Like I'm gonna spend money when I look like this?"

I was perplexed. She'd fallen sanely and mutually in love. He had known and loved her fat and thin and had asked her to marry him when she was at seventy-five pounds into her regain.

"So?" I asked. "You still ought to dress up."

"Fff't."

I'm a clothes whore and would never pass up a chance to get dressed up—if only I hadn't developed a panic disorder that, when it came to the afternoon of B.J.'s party, erupted in a full-blown meltdown of hyperventilation and hysteria because I hadn't taken a Klonopin. One of the costs of B.J.'s weight gain was pretty party clothes. One of my costs was parties.

Fat acceptance adherents and fat dieters are equally at odds with a world we don't fit and a public that claims the right to judge us. One afternoon just after my birthday celebration with Mimi, I was walking nonagenarian Zeke, a pony-sized Lab/Great Dane mix with the spirit and wisdom of Lao-tzu. As we paused to consider which way to go, an aging Indian woman, hurrying to the subway, stopped to look at us. She said something I didn't understand but took to refer to the arthritic gentle giant at my side. I wrinkled my eyebrows trying to pick apart her rush of words and shook my head in confusion.

"U-ee-mow-ves-yo-sck-gaw-dn?" she repeated.

I shook my head. "I'm sorry. I don't understand."

She smiled and continued on her way to the Seventh Avenue train. I looked at Zeke trying to make out what she had said about him. It hit me, then: "You eat more vegetables, your stomach will go down."

The woman wasn't exactly skinny—she was kind of plump, as far as I could tell. It was frosty and she was wearing a heavy jacket. She had given her advice with a sweetness that wasn't, almost, offensive.

We don't wear badges proclaiming our weight loss or our plans; few people know that we're "doing something about it" and that we want to be granted some immunity from well-meaning strangers and the self-righteous. We are still objects of assumptions, still looking for something fabulous to wear to the Christmas office party, still having to use our fat bodies to run a library or do the laundry or take a swim class. But because we have a different future body in mind, we dieters of size live in a netherworld. We are fat, but we aren't Fat.

To be Fat is to think about fat in the broadest terms at all times. Fat becomes an asset, an example, and an achievement. "Now that I weigh 270 pounds and have friends twice my size, I realize that this numbers game is no different from the flat-world theory," Marilyn Wann crows in *Fat!So?*[76]

To celebrate one's fat as the "essence" of one's self, couched in terms of achievement, is as exclusionary as Mimi thinking of her fat as a character fault. NAAFA's glorying in pulchritude is fat-minded, fat-oriented, fat-informed, fat-defensive, fat-social, fat-professional. Ultimately, it can become a dogma and a cult.

To be fair, dieters aren't immune from this corporeal gestalt. If we were, we wouldn't be part of a thriving blogging world in which we share stories, progress, backsliding, confusions, and philosophies. Points, calories, ounces, pounds lost and pounds to lose, threshold weights, days of abstinence, clothing sizes, minutes on the rowing machine, miles biked, keychains, magnets, coins: it is difficult not to obsess.

Further, with the publication of my first book, I found myself expected to be professionally thin. Identifying myself by my clothing size, writing and talking about it, and having my publisher, agent, and publicists hoping that I would approach the star value of Oprah, Kirstie Alley, the Duchess of Windsor, Al Roker, Carnie Wilson, Lynn Redgrave, and Valerie Bertinelli is one of the aspects of going back to the planet of girls that I do not want to live again.

Unlike the stars, I don't tout a weight-loss method, nor does anyone in the diet blogging world the Angry Fat Girls inhabit, even though each us has a plan and an allegiance that works, or that we want to work, for us. Fat people are welcome, whether they are dieting or not. Fat acceptance proponents are welcome. Their insights and experiences are invaluable because every woman has a fat girl inside her.

---

76   Marilyn Wann, *Fat!So?* (Berkeley, Ten Speed Press, 1998), 29.

If an active NAAFA or HAES member would speak frankly with me, I would want to know if she has lived Katie's, Wendy's, Mimi's, and my experiences of obesity. Has she ever been so big that she had to use an instrument with which to wipe her ass? Has she had to place a stool in her shower? Has she had to sleep sitting up? Has she developed arthritis from the weight she's carried? Has she ever been on disability because she could no longer hoist her body from bed to work?

Does she accept these conditions with serenity?

I would want to know if the spokesperson I was speaking to could bend over to tie her shoes, if she missed having an enveloping hug. I'd want to know what her level of fear or dread was of going to get a haircut and sitting in the foot-pumped chair, of going to the doctor, of receiving a necklace as a gift, of a ninety-degree day when the humidity was so high that the horizon was the color of weak milky tea.

Because I consider these to be voluntary roadblocks, rather than immutable facts. And they get in the way of living in a certain kind of freedom.

Thankfully, not all fat acceptance writers are at complete peace with their decision to stop dieting. When I asked Maureen Wood, who writes the Large & Lovely Site for BellaOnline, how she has learned to accept and embrace being fat, she responded, "I don't think I am at 'peace' with my body. Sometimes I feel like a fraud telling women and young girls they have a right to be who they are and feel good about themselves when I'm constantly battling my own demons, but I honestly want them to believe it because that's the way it should be. I come from the frame of reference [that] if you keep telling yourself (and everyone else) it's so, then one day it will be so."

After reading Wendy Shanker's *The Fat Girl's Guide to Life* and Lara Frater's *Fat Chicks Rule!*, I was relieved when each reported days on which they look in the mirror and shudder at their size, and that size acceptance is a process rather than a decision like turning on a lamp. Both women, who are in the thirties, come from backgrounds of iron-woman dieting and they understand the desire to be thin. "People have free will." Lara says. "They feel they can lose weight. But please don't lecture me on weight, and don't pitch your diet to me."They have settled at stable weights in what the medical world calls Obesity Class 1, and they have maintained their weights for a number of years. They eat correctly, they exercise, their vital statistics are normal. Frater and Shanker are evidence that support NAAFA's citations of the thirty-year-old works of William Bennet, MD, and Paul Ernsberger, PhD. The new millennium has at last brought another voice, Paul Campos, PhD, to the discussion of whether obesity is overrated as a health problem in the United States and whether fitness is more important than body mass.

Stable and healthy as writers like Frater may be, fat acceptance and HAES mouthpieces break down in defensiveness and resentment. Anger and blame (on fashion designers, the media, the scientific and medical community, loved ones, the diet industry, the thin, family, the past) are rife in the fat-positive world:

I knew it was not concern for my health when my husband of more than four decades grabbed a bag of potato chips from my hand, which he and one of our daughters were sharing as we watched a video at midnight on New Year's Eve, 1995. He expressed disgust that I continued to eat potato chips after he had stopped. Lamely, through terrible hurt feelings, I told him he was not in charge of what I ate. "I guess not!" he yelled, an unmistakable reference that if he were, I would look different.[77]

It would seem that, in choosing between trying to lose weight or working toward acceptance of one's fat, one has to decide, among

---

77 Frater, 12.

other things, whether she wants to be pissed off at herself or pissed off at the world.

Mimi was pissed off when she moved back to Philadelphia in 1990. She planned her move carefully, the way Mimi does everything. This time it included joining Nutrisystem and losing seventy pounds in the eight months before she settled into her office in the Johnson Pavilion. She weighed 220 pounds—a haunting number—but in her growing fury over what happened in North Carolina, she didn't really care. After seeing a small ad in a neighborhood newspaper, she consulted a therapist who specialized in treating women who have been sexually abused by men in power. Within fifteen minutes of listening to Mimi's story, Lena Nord told her that Michael Clark was not only a textbook abuser, but probably a serial one at that.

Under Lena's tutelage, Mimi went to her local diocese and initiated the process of seeking redress. "I couldn't watch my weight and go through all of that," she says. "I had to write out exactly what happened and it took forty-five pages. Then I reduced it to a summary of two pages. I didn't say a word to my bishop when I met with him. I just handed him the document and waited for him to read it.

"I should have learned not to trust men," she says of the saga. She weighed 270 pounds when she left therapy. Waiting around for the new life that settling the past and talk therapy had promised took two years and added another forty pounds.

That's when she was lured into 1 Enoch, a West Philadelphia bookstore, in search of inspiration.

The store had a large plate-glass window framed in rainbow-painting prisms. Prominently displayed was a plump iron pot brimming with daffodils. There were books on gardening, cooking, and meditation. Ropes of whole spices hung in the background; she recognized cinnamon sticks and nutmeg and star anise, and her nose twitched at what the shop must smell like. Forming an arc around the flowers were cracked quartzes in rose and yellow and minty green. Mimi felt her shoulder blades flex and relax as she studied the window. Her breath slowed and deepened. She badly wanted to hold the pale green quartz against her cheek.

It smelled of licorice inside. A tea urn sent up a thin steam of it. She helped herself to a cup and held it in both hands, loving the heat after the windy March evening. She studied the books and lingered over the shelves of spices and herbs—many of which she'd never heard of, rows of candles in primary colors, a collection of sand dollars, jars of salt and sand, and piles of delicious velvet swatches and silk cords.

As she leafed through a Moosewood cookbook that made her shake her head in dismay at all the cheese and carbohydrates it called for, she felt an arm slide along her shoulder. Another book appeared in front of her, glossy with leafy greens and a proclamation in red that it would teach its user to "eat for life." A dark, long-fingered hand held it.

"You might like this," a baritone Jamaican voice said.

Mimi turned and faced a tall, thin man, so dark that his face glinted blue under the natural sunlamps spaced over the bookshelves. His hair was in dreadlocks that reached his butt, tied back with a long white cord. He smiled and his face lit like dawn.

"You're a Cancer, aren't you? I can always tell by the way you find the designs in the seashells and then end up at the cookbooks. I'm Sleight," he added.

Mimi looked perplexed.

He laughed. "Not slight as in small. That would be you." He beamed down from his great height. "Sleight as in magic. Sleight as in"—he took the Moosewood cookbook from her and restocked it on the shelf—"deft of hand."

She was enchanted.

"I'm Mimi," she answered, and marveled at how calm her voice was.

"Of course. Let me pour you another cup of tea, and we can get to know each other." He nodded to two worn, comfy-looking purple velvet club chairs angled at a coffee table covered in magazines and pamphlets. "Anise is purifying and increases your psychic power. We can talk more about that."

If she thought getting free of Michael Clark was hard, she was about to go through four years of "apprenticeship" to a man she gave her destiny to, a man who took it and, too soon, forgot he had it.

The clues to her future were everywhere.

Enoch is a book excluded from the Old Testament by everyone except for the Ethiopian Orthodox Church. The number 1 refers to the only complete copy, which is written in Ethiopic, and the book, a cross between the fall of the Titans and the Book of Revelation, is a vision of end times given by God to Enoch, the grandfather of Noah, about the angels who dared mate with human women and the violence and necromancy they wreaked upon the earth.

The real name of the owner of 1 Enoch was Morris Johns but he went by Sleight to everyone but his bank and the IRS. Three weeks later, when he invited Mimi into the circle cast in celebration of the reunion of Persephone and Demeter, he was Samyaza, the angel who led two hundred angels to copulate with the daughters of man.

Mimi asked to be apprenticed to his coven. He agreed gladly and was only a little less hesitant when she asked to be his apprentice. "I need to be led," she told him.

"You need to be taught," he countered. "You don't know enough of the Ways to know I am your teacher."

"I know you," she answered, and he agreed to tutor her in the spells and rituals of the coven known as the Watchers—those angels who left heaven to create a race of giants on earth.

"There was so much that was good there," Mimi says of her four years, "but Sleight was one of those priests who's in it for superstardom. It was all about being the biggest group with the most specialties and the most public celebrations. We regularly met up at Rittenhouse

Square or Longwood Gardens to chant and dance and hand out leaf-
lets for 1 Enoch and neo-paganism. Sleight had a dozen apprentices
and none of us went through the three lunar cycles of training and
the year-and-a-day initiation that is customary for apprentices to go
through. We were in and anything we learned beyond the basics, like
casting a circle and calling the quarters, we learned on our own or
from someone else."

Among the basics that Sleight used in his pamphlets and introductory remarks were the two official laws of Wicca. The first two of
these rules come from the Rede, the governing code for all practitioners of white magick: "An' ye harm none, do what ye will" and the
Threefold Law, "All good that a person does to another returns threefold in this life; harm is also returned threefold."

Sleight's third rule is from the turn-of-the-century *Gospel of the
Witches*. It is a subject of much discussion among Wiccans and his
employment of it bore his twist on the craft:

> *And as the sign that ye are truly free
> Ye shall be naked in your rites, both men
> And women also . . .*

Sleight's rules for Mimi were that she serve and obey him, and
that she fall in love with him.

That had already happened, when he offered her the alternative
cookbook, three weeks before the vernal equinox and the rites of
Ostara and its promises of new beginnings with the advent of spring.

Mimi redesigned the Watchers' website and monitored their active
posts, editing out anything that might displease Sleight. He praised
her work, praised her prettiness, and urged her to explore her goddess connection. She had her hair colored, took makeup lessons, and
bought more striking clothes. And she got interested in herbs, turning
to Jolene, a.k.a. Sky Gull, a former apprentice to Sleight. Jolene didn't
show up often for gatherings, and never for public ones. She hinted

at things about herbs and spices, waxes and colors, that Sleight didn't know, that could protect their user from harm close at hand. Mimi thought of Sleight's long hands and said no one could know everything and asked about the uses of lemon peel.

When you are mesmerized—by a man or a project, a successful diet or research or friend—time flows in too-quick starts and relentless stops. In March of 2002, confident that Sleight would mystically guide her through the weight-loss process, Mimi left Weight Watchers. She paid little attention to what she was snacking on through the day and at night, curled up in her La-Z-Boy while she read and wrote in the leather grimoire she bought at 1 Enoch. It came as a shock when she had to spend a night in the Penn Sleep Center for a radical adjustment of her CPAP machine and saw that she had drifted up to 340 pounds in the two years since she met Sleight.

"Is it because of my weight?" she asked the pulmonologist after he explained that she'd gone from twenty to twenty-five breathing pauses per hour to thirty to forty.

"I can't say whether it is or it isn't," he answered. "Thin people have sleep apnea, too. What I can say is that the obese are far more prone to the condition, and your events absolutely wouldn't get worse if you lose weight, while they very might get worse if you gain more."

It was back to Weight Watchers again—and it was back to discussing her food and eating with a man as her spiritual advisor. In the next two years she lost more than 104 pounds, the only time she has crossed the 211-pound barrier.

Sex with a priest can be very inspiring, especially one who has the psychic power to lend strength of will to a beloved.

Until, that is, the beloved finds out she is *one* of the beloved, one of the *old* beloved, and in fact, has been led to be regarded by the *new* circle of women around Sleight as a pain in the ass.

Mimi was so much a pain in the ass—showing up for gatherings, going to Sleight's scarily barren apartment when he called in the middle of the night, running the website—that Sleight sent Jenny (a.k.a. Brighid) to her office with a letter saying she was banned from the coven and was never to contact Samyaza again.

How much do eight million tears weigh?

The story of Sleight was an open-ended denouement because she had a friend in Jolene who could confirm Sleight's habit of picking up and dropping women, and who encouraged her to practice her Craft on her own and to make contact with other solitary practitioners. Still, Mimi has bumped around the scale more than any of the rest of us, and each high she reaches before getting into another serious course of Weight Watchers has a history of grief.

Mimi finished telling me the cautionary tale of Sleight as we waited for her train back to Philadelphia. We lucked out and found two seats, and were surrounded by bags that included jokey Christmas gifts for Katie, Lindsay, and Wendy. We'd found the perfect booth in Union Square that had a variety of grow-your-own fill-in-the-blank items. A boyfriend for Wendy, a personal trainer for Lindsay, a shrink for Katie. I had learned a lot about Mimi that day that I loved— her delight in taking pictures, which I share, her perfect window-shopping sensibility, the source of her compassion for Wendy, and a peek into her iconography (Green Man images, tasteful fat ladies, fat smiling suns, and flying pigs, which were another thing we liked in common).

"So why do you put yourself through it all?" I asked. "You're at Penn School of Medicine, for Christ's sake. Look at the new findings on all the obesity scare stories. You're pretty, funny, so smart, kind, talented, professional—being thin isn't going to enhance that, and it's not going to cure your arthritis. You've joined water aerobics to get more fit, which is so cool. Why not . . . give up?"

"Because," she snapped, "I will never give my body 'up' again. Not to a man, not to a group, not to food. I may not be in charge yet, but I'm working on it. *I* get to be the boss of me, and I want the strength and discipline I get from losing weight to help do all that bossing."

So there it was. Mimi wanted sovereignty over her body in order to own her life, whether it meant obeying or rebelling against a food plan. Her train was announced, and we gathered our stuff and walked to the train. Hours earlier, I'd sneaked back to the seller of handblown Polish ornaments to buy her a Louis Comfort Tiffany ball that I gave her at the gate.

She smiled lovingly at the delicate blue, green, and yellow reproduction of the dragonflies and folded the box back up before hugging me. "Good-bye, Francie," she said. "Thank you for asking me to spend this day with you."

"And thank you for coming. I love you, Meems."

"I love you, too," she said, and hugged me again.

She'd found my family nickname intuitively, and I knew that, this time, the return "I love you" was sincere.

January
Unfun Facts to Know and Tell

Wherever the Angry Fat Girls were on New Year's Day of 2007, it was unnaturally warm. "There's snowdrops on campus," Wendy told me when she called me in Arizona to see how I was faring after I posted a desperate description on my personal blog. One of Wendy's MOs is to offer a story or newspaper article as consolation for an entirely different crisis. Mimi also called but asked more direct questions as I lay on my parents' couch with the Christmas tree for company and sobbed about cookies and old age and boredom and Scott and pie.

"Can you go to bed without eating tonight?" she asked.

"Maybe," I sniveled.

"Can you drink eight glasses of water a day until you get back? Just do one thing from your food plan, okay, sweetie?"

"Better," I said as I carried the phone and another pile of cookies into my bedroom, grateful that my father was blind and my mother slept more and more as her heart weakened. "How are you?" It was best to move away from my slightly gray lie to whatever had poked Wendy to dial my parents' house.

"Ah'm all right, Ah guess . . . Ah'm lookin' at all the women on Match.com to see what they say about themselves. Ah just don' think Ah can claim bein' outdoorsy, do you?"

I laughed. "How were *your* parents over Christmas?"

"I bought my mom a blouse for two dollars, which she loved and tried to give back to me." She gave one of her cackling laughs that cats save for going into heat. I held the phone away from my ear until she finished. "Now I'm about ready to drive down to Hillsville and yell at my mother 'cause she's callin' me and sayin' stupid shit like, 'I hope you're not depressed' 'cause Ah'm not with Leo and Ah don' have a boyfriend for new year. It's almost like she's not happy unless I cry and say, 'I wish I were dead.'"

Where did I read that banging your head against a wall burns 150 calories an hour?

"Got any resolutions?" I asked as I fed a piece of peanut butter cookie to Daisy.

"Ah'm thinkin' about takin' tennis lessons. I wonder what the other girls are plannin'?"

Mimi emailed me an answer to that question the next day. She'd been in upstate New York, at a reading of *The Golden Bough*. She was hoping *this* would be the year she got to a comfortable weight. In San Bruno, California, Katie emailed about which futility she should settle on—lose weight? stop overreacting to life? stay out of her family's quarrels?—as she tried to teach Apple and Orange, her kittens, not to climb the curtains, where they would be seen by her pet-phobic landlords. I avoid New Year's resolutions, but that was the year I was forced to finally concede that Scott hurt me more than he comforted or supported me.

New Year's Day meant a gathering of the Longhetti clan at Lindsay's uncle Ted's house in Barberton, just south of Akron. Lindsay adored Uncle Ted, a retired battalion chief of the Akron Fire Department. He was her father's identical twin, and the two men finished each other's jokes, swore in the same language at the stupidity of the Browns quarterbacks, and had worked together to build extensions and swimming pools at each other's home and the cabin in Upper Sandusky, tinkering at whatever engines came their way. Her parents and sisters would be there and so would her cousins Jilly and Terri. That was the good news. The bad news was that this was also Aunt Carol's house. The Aunt Carol who always had a dig at her weight and her sisters' and cousins' lack thereof.

"Please don't just stand there when Aunt Carol asks what kind of goodies I ate at Christmas," she asked Jalen as she left the interstate for Wooster Road. "If she mentions that Jilly had to take all her Christmas presents back because they were too big—"

Her sentence hung. What could Jalen do? Smack Carol? Wonder aloud if Jilly had an eating disorder? Ask Aunt Carol where her daughter got the thin genes?

"—ask where Jilly got her thin genetics or something, okay?" Aunt Carol looked a lot like Aunt Bea in *The Andy Griffith Show* and Uncle Ted, like her dad, had a belly that made summer swim parties a hoot because it kept popping out of his trunks. But whereas Dean Longhetti fought his gut fat, Uncle Ted laughed along with them at it and only shrugged when he'd been diagnosed with diabetes a couple of years ago.

And so, the moment she saw Uncle Ted barefoot at the door, she was furious at herself for wearing clogs without socks.

She nudged Jalen and nodded at his feet.

"What did the doctor tell you about going barefoot? Where's your cane?" Lindsay asked.

"And happy New Year to you, too, Linny," he said.

"Unc," Lindsay said with a note of warning in her voice.

"I'm in the house, for Christ's sake," he said. "My shoe feels funny."

Back in September, Lindsay had heard on the Longhetti grape-vine how Ted stepped on a piece of glass when he was winterizing the pool. It wasn't until Aunt Carol saw brown spots on her white carpet that evening that he noticed the cut. Despite a thorough cleaning and daily changes of dressings, Lindsay's mom told her, the cut turned nastier by Halloween. Lindsay drove over to check Uncle Ted out for herself. She heard the uneven footsteps of someone limping in pain before he answered the door.

"I'm hearing rumors," she said with both hands on her hips. "I want to see the cut."

He winced as he turned toward the living room, then covered the intake with a laugh. "It's Halloween, Linny-girl. It's my God-given costume."

"Just because you've been Santa for the toy drive every year since Jesus was born doesn't mean you get to maim yourself for every holiday," she retorted. She knelt down and pulled off his sock, then unwound the gauze. She felt faint from the strong smell of ferment-ing yeast. The flesh was peeling and a palm-sized area around the joint of the big toe was hot to the touch. Lindsay pulled out her cell phone and called her dad to come take Uncle Ted to the doctor. He ended up in the hospital for a night of intravenous antibiotics before the doc would debride the widening hole between the toe and foot.

Aunt Carol was a guilty wreck that she hadn't taken it more seriously, so Lindsay's dad was there when they got to speak to the physician. The news was bad. The infection was eating into the ten-don. Uncle Ted went back every week to have the wound cleaned and inspected. He was warned at the end of every treatment about using his cane and wearing shoes. The swelling had burst blood ves-sels, and his foot and ankle turned a spidery purple and black. Worse, Uncle Ted's moods, which had been dependably serious or jolly all of Lindsay's life, alternated between defensiveness and whining within the same sentence, which was what scared her most. She wanted her uncle, the muscled, gregarious guy who could install a swimming pool, change the oil on her Mazda, and then round up the Longhettis for touch football after dinner.

"Aunt Carol said she got you size-fourteen sneakers for Christmas," Lindsay lectured.

"It's like walking on skis," he said. "Give an old man a break, Linny. It doesn't matter anyway."

She bit her tongue to keep from saying it most certainly *did* matter. The dressing slid around when he walked barefoot. Without feeling in his feet, he was frightened of slipping in socks, and he resisted leaving the house because of the ugly swelling and bizarre footwear. His complexion was pasty, and he looked soft from lack of activity.

Lindsay poked Jalen. "I want you to show Uncs some things he can do with hand weights and a resistance tube. You need to get him moving."

Jalen nodded. Exercise is both Jalen's and Lindsay's answer to everything—exercise and following her orders. Ted had already had a battery of cardiologists, endocrinologists, and orthopedists giving him clear instructions about how to manage his heart, diabetes, and infection, but it was Jalen who could help him get some strength back.

Her cousin Terri was sitting at the table tearing salad greens as her mother and Aunt Carol peeled potatoes. "I'm worried sick," Carol was saying, "but I can't watch him all the time. He's sixty years old, not a toddler."

Lindsay kissed everyone hello and took a wineglass from the dozen on the counter. "You guys talking about Unc not wearing shoes?"

The silence made Lindsay look at Aunt Carol closely. Her mouth was trembling, and Terri started slashing the salad spinner as though mustering troops to battle.

"What's going on?" she asked. Aunt Carol looked at Terri.

"There's been a . . . complication," she said.

"What complication? With Uncle Ted's foot? His heart? What?" Lindsay asked.

"His foot. Dr. Stetts says it's wet gangrene. The infection is eating into the bone."

Lindsay sat down, hard, on the nearest chair. "When did you find this out?"

"Yesterday. I could see the color had changed to yellow, and I called Terri and your dad. We took him to the emergency room, and Dr. Stetts had him stay overnight. They debrided more but . . . they're going to have to take his foot off."

"Why didn't you call us?" Lindsay looked from her aunt to her mother, who shook her head in defeat. "I would have come up. I would have talked to Dr. Stetts. There have to be other therapies."

"He's had double-bypass surgery, so his circulation is not all that good. There wasn't anything you could have done to keep this from happening."

Lindsay returned her glare to her mother. "There has to be something we can do."

As the Longhettis ate their New Year's dinner of ham, scalloped potatoes, steamed green beans, salad, dinner rolls and I Can't Believe It's Not Butter, hot fruit salad, and vanilla ice cream, seven metabolisms launched into the same chain of events. The masticated green beans entered the stomach, the temporary holding area for food, which shrinks to hold a quarter of a cup of liquid when empty and can swell to about eight and a half pints after a heavy meal. The stomach produces and secretes gastric acids and digestive enzymes that break down the ham from large molecules into the small ones that can be passed into the small intestine, a process that takes forty minutes to a few hours.

Most of the nutrients from the New Year's Day meal the Longhettis shared were extracted in the duodenum, the first section of the twenty-foot tube of the small intestine. The presence of proteins and fats in the duodenum prompts the secretions of hormones that alert the pancreas to release the pancreatic juice that will help to neutralize acids along with a number of enzymes that break down fats into lipids, proteins into amino acids, and starch into glucose, the body's main source of cellular fuel. These secretions are half of the pancreas's job.

I doubt that Lindsay's family would have found this fitting conversation as they ate a tense dinner while not mentioning Ted's upcoming amputation. But to understand, or reinterpret, the establishment hype about obesity, diabetes type 2, dietary and exercise requirements, bariatric surgery, hormone experiments, and other matters fat people have to consider on a daily basis, it's essential to have a course in Metabolism 101.

The second job the pancreas performs is in the production of insulin. Insulin is a hormone (that is, a messenger cell) that, after Ted Longhetti finished his salad, tells and allows the liver, muscles, and fat to absorb glucose in order to keep the blood glucose level.

The Longhettis' new army of insulin had another, overlooked effect on their metabolisms: it coalesces fatty acids into triglycerides, which, as clumps of fatty acids, couldn't enter the body's cells, which were feasting on glucose. Those triglycerides retreated into the adipose tissue that is Ted's potbelly. Increased insulin makes us store fat. In *Good Calories, Bad Calories*, Gary Taubes directly confronts the ongoing orthodoxy of counting calories while following a low-fat diet. "It is important also to know that the fat cells of adipose tissue are 'exquisitely sensitive' to insulin . . . Elevating insulin even slightly will increase the accumulation of fat in the cells. The longer insulin remains elevated, the longer the fat cells will accumulate fat, and the longer they'll go without releasing it."[78]

As Uncle Ted shuffled off with his brother and sons-in-law to catch the kickoff, too many of his blood cells did not recognize the insulin that was trying to open doors for the new glucose to be stored

---

78 Gary Taubes, *Good Calories, Bad Calories: Challenging the Conventional Wisdom on Diet, Weight Control, and Disease* (New York: Alfred A. Knopf, 2007), 393.

for later use. Lindsay's push to get her uncle exercising was correct: by getting his muscles in shape, he would be able to break down his glucose better. Without medication, careful diet, and exercise, his blood can overload with glucose, which can eventually lead to diseased blood vessels—diabetic angiopathy.

Ted Longhetti has type 2 diabetes mellitus and is insulin resistant. While he produces enough insulin for a nondiabetic, his body is desensitized, inhibiting his muscle cells from absorbing the glucose they need. At the same time, his liver goes into overdrive to produce yet more glucose, thus glutting his blood with more glucose than it can use and effectively starving his body. Type 2 diabetes is the most common form of diabetes, affecting about 2,780,000 Americans, or just over one-sixth of the population.[79] More than one-tenth of men who are twenty years and older—10.9 million—have type 2 diabetes mellitus, while nearly one-ninth or 9.7 million women in the same age group suffer from the disease. Another 54 million people are prediabetic, a condition in which blood glucose is higher than normal.

New diagnoses peak in the forty to fifty-nine age group. Diabetes (and its complications) is the sixth leading cause of death in the United States, and its annual costs are $92 billion in medical care and another $40 billion in premature death, disability, and job losses. Consider that from 1995 to 2005, the Department of Agriculture spent $51.3 billion in corn subsidies (which kept a low ceiling on the cost of high fructose corn syrup, a suspicious substance in the story of type 2 diabetes). The drain on diabetics' (and insurers' and taxpayers') wallets is something like a national emergency.

In 2003, Lindsay's uncle was diagnosed as having been diabetic for a number of years. He'd been complaining of being thirsty and

---

79   According to the American Diabetes Association, 7 percent of the American population is diabetic. The figures I've given exempt type 1 and gestational diabetes.

having prickly feet. The family's confusion stemmed from the fact that he didn't look like someone who is diabetic.

"It's not like he's fat," Lindsay had said to her cousin Jilly as they sat on the patio watching Jalen and Jilly's husband, Peter, scrapping in the pool. "He's not obese. Up until he hurt himself, he was always busy around the house or fixing cars or going up to the cabin."

The term *type 2 diabetes* is a fairly recent one. The disease used to be known as non-insulin-dependent diabetes, adult-onset diabetes, and, originally, obese diabetes. The traditional association of obesity and diabetes is a tie as strong as the umbilical cord and, in fact, 55 percent of people suffering from type 2 diabetes are obese.[80] If you read the barrage of antiobesity warnings, you'll see that diabetes is at the top of the list of obesity-caused diseases. These warnings do not differentiate between overweight and obese, and they do not educate the public in the kinds of fat that make up both of those categories.

Lindsay was also right in that Ted wasn't in need of a bariatric chair (that is, a chair designed for a four-hundred-or-more-pound body), but like a lot of men he was prone to a beer gut. Extensive studies have shown that an apple-shaped body is at a much greater risk for diabetes and clogged arteries, heart disease, and female cancers. Men are generally apple shaped (as am I, dammit), and this is reflected in the genders' different statistics. Belly fat, known as visceral or deep fat,[81] collects and releases the fatty acids into the bloodstream, where

---

80 M. S. Eberhart, C. Ogden, M. Engelau, B. Cadwell, A. A. Hedley, S. H. Saydah, "Prevalence of Overweight and Obesity among Adults with Diagnosed Diabetes: United States 1988–1994 and 1999–2002: The standards outlined," *Morbidity and Mortality Weekly Report, Centers for Disease Control and Prevention* 53, no. 45 (November 19, 2004): 1066–68.

81 The other two types of body fat are intramuscular fat, which veins skeletal muscles, and the subcutaneous fat under the skin, the fat we curse on our thighs and buttocks.

they can clog arteries and interfere with the belly's neighbor, the liver, which can result in higher insulin levels.[82]

Lindsay's concern was bolstered by the strong heritability factor for obesity, and for glucose and insulin levels that can result in type 2 diabetes. Fourteen percent of children will develop type 2 diabetes if one parent is diagnosed before the age of fifty; if the parent is diagnosed after fifty, the number hovers just under 8 percent. If both parents are diagnosed, at any age, their children will have a 50 percent chance of developing the disease.[83]

Uncle Ted's genes are identical to Lindsay's father's. She could be that one-in-seven offspring to get sick. These statistics are one of Lindsay's reasons for wanting to lose weight and maintain an exercise schedule. She has done the waist-to-hip tabulation that can give a general sense of the risk of metabolic disorders and was relieved, for a change, that she is pear shaped.[84] But relative risks and preventative measures were not on Lindsay's mind on January seventeenth when the doctors kept her father, aunt, and cousins waiting all day for news on how Uncle Ted's amputation surgery went.

Eight hours after he was wheeled into the OR, the Longhettis were finally informed that the surgery went well and were allowed to

---

82   Glenn A. Gaesser, *Big Fat Lies: The Truth about Your Weight and Your Health* (New York: Ballantine, 1996), 130–33.

83   James Gavin, "Diabetes Onset: A combination of genes & environmental influences," http://www.isletsofhope.com (accessed).

84   "Use a tape measure to measure the circumference of your waist at its smallest point—usually just above your navel. A waist measurement of greater than 40 inches (102 centimeters) for men or 35 inches (89 centimeters) for women indicates increased health risks [i.e., coronary disease, diabetes, ovarian/prostate/testicular cancers]. Use a tape measure to measure the circumference of your waist at its smallest point. Then measure the circumference of your hips at their widest point. To calculate your waist-to-hip ratio, divide your waist measurement by your hip measurement. A waist-to-hip ratio of greater than 0.9 for men and 0.85 for women indicates increased health risks." Martha Grogan, MD, http://mayoclinic.com (accessed).

see him. They were surprised to find he was uncharacteristically cranky. He was in pain and he was scared of being moved from the hospital to a rehabilitation facility where he would be fitted with a prosthesis and undergo the initial physical therapy that would allow him to go home. "I'm a cripple," he kept saying. "What can a cripple do?" Lindsay took a deep breath and began a mental list of the inspirational stories she would assemble for him, the exercise plan she would get Jalen to go over and do every day with him, the support groups she would find and get Aunt Carol to attend with him.

The situation was a call for action and, in a way, Lindsay was grateful for that. Action—research, questions, plans, therapies, sources, outcomes—is Lindsay's specialty. Just as Jalen's exercise addiction required therapy and group support, and her own rah-rah insistence that he get help mandated that she learn how not to indulge him, Lindsay needed forward motion in order to feel that life was taking place. Part of her success in balancing a nervy husband, graduate school, work, a home, and her big family and Jalen's, too, was that Lindsay didn't dwell on what she couldn't do. She couldn't go to Yale? Then go to Kent State. She couldn't stand apartments? Plop a down payment on a house and not only stick to the savings plan but don't be ashamed to pick up pennies on the street. That philosophy was what would rescue Uncle Ted. His depression would lift when they mapped out a recovery plan, got him exercising, got him interested in what he *could* do—hand weights, swimming, wall push-ups—instead of what he couldn't do.

Which amounted to, after time and physical therapy, eat a sheet cake or walk barefoot.

Unfortunately, while Ted Longhetti and his doctors could take measures to treat his diabetes, the nearly canonical recommendations for prevention and treatment leave the Angry Fat Girls with as many questions as precepts.

Does weighing four hundred pounds cause insulin deficiency, or do some pancreases produce only enough insulin for, say, a weight of two hundred pounds?

How carefully has that 55 percent of obese diabetics been vetted for having diabetes in their family, for their lifestyles before and after diagnosis? Is it weight loss that brings blood sugar into manageable range, or is it the change of lifestyle? How many healthy obese people (that is to say, people who eat their vegetables, limit their cheesecake, don't smoke, and get an hour of exercise in every day) develop the disease?

That January, Katie resolved to make her case to her insurance provider for gastric bypass surgery. She'd spent nine months jumping through their hoops, and she felt 2007 belonged to her. Katie describes her body as the "Big Apple," and after falling off her summer food plan on which she'd gone from 427 to 398 pounds, she was as round as ever. She ate her way through the four-fecta of witch-shaped cakes, turkey-shaped cakes, Christmas tree cakes, and glittery happy New Year cakes, and then some. After all, on November first, the jack-o'-lantern chocolate cakes with orange frosting and licorice whip grins were one-third the price that they were the day before.

There's almost nothing worse that we bakery-lovers could love. Not all sugars are created equal. There has been a great deal of talk in the media and nutrition circles about the perils of high fructose corn syrup, what Martha Beck calls "the sweat of Satan."[85] In the last thirty years it has gained preeminence as a sweetener because of its long shelf life. With corn plentiful and cheap, cane, fruit, and beet sugars fell out of commercial usage, but high fructose corn syrup is as different from those other sugars as aspirin is from heroin. Fructose

---

85   Martha Beck, *The Four Day Win: End Your Diet War and Achieve Thinner Peace* (New York: Rodale, 2008), 2.

metabolizes straight to the liver and apes insulin by releasing triglycerides that lead to high cholesterol and atherosclerosis.[86]

Katie and I were the smokers among the AFGs, and any conversation with her was interrupted with a shouted order for "large Diet Coke with lots of ice" or "Venti latte with skim milk, please." We were also the two AFGs under psychiatric supervision for anxiety and mood disorders. Alcohol, tobacco, caffeine, and stress portend hypoglycemia as much as sugar does, and yet, as Katie met with surgeons and shrinks that January, her blood sugar and blood pressure were within normal range.

She might have gotten closer to the operating room had she been prediabetic or diabetic. A four-year study conducted by the University Obesity Research Center in Australia found that of the sixty obese, diabetic patients who were either assigned to a diet-and-exercise system or had laparoscopic adjustable gastric bypass, 73 percent of the surgical patients had diabetic remission, while 13 percent in the lifestyle control group experienced remission. After two years, the surgical patients lost 20 percent of their body weight and the control group under 2 percent.

The study, published in *The Journal of the American Medical Association* in January 2008, showed up in headlines around the world, each more misleading than the next: "Weight Loss Surgery Helps Treat Diabetes," "Weight Loss Surgery Can Send Diabetics into Remission," "Stomach Bands a Diabetes Fix," "Obesity Surgery Can Cure Diabetes." How many diabetics opened up their morning papers to be greeted with a moment's promise that, somehow, the adjustable

---

86   Fructose is found in honey, many berries, true fruits, some root vegetables (sweet potatoes, parsnips, beets, and onions), usually combined with glucose. The digestive system also manufactures fructose from table sugar (sucrose). Sucrose is the combination of fructose and glucose. Jack Challem, "Fructose: Maybe Not So Natural . . . and Not So Safe," *The Nutrition Reporter* (1995).

gastric Lap-Band would cure them? Even the authors of the *JAMA* editorial were extremely cautious about the efficacy of the surgery: "Participants randomized to surgical therapy were more likely to achieve remission of type 2 diabetes through greater weight loss. These results need to be confirmed in a larger, more diverse population and have long-term efficacy assessed."[87] Still, the authors beg the question of whether it was weight loss or the extreme shift in lifestyle that resolved the patients' diabetes.

In any case, with the American Society for Metabolic and Bariatric Surgery reporting 220,000 weight-loss surgeries performed in the United States in 2008,[88] the number will only increase if the surgery is perceived to be a means of controlling diabetes.

And yet Katie, at 409 pounds, was turned down for gastric bypass surgery, for the second time, by Kaiser Permanente. She was in a towering rage.

Through her dialectical behavior classes, with the help of the therapist referred by her insurance provider, she was tutored in reacting to events and situations less hastily and less emotively. For a long time, the heading on her blog was a quote from Don Miguel Ruiz's *The Four Agreements*: "Don't take anything personally." Ruiz's admonition and the dialectical behavior skills she was schooled in were precepts she wanted to live up to rather than rules she managed to live by. It's ironic, then, that one of her worst breakdowns started on a rainy Tuesday in January when she talked to her new therapist, the pre-weight-loss-surgery evaluator, about how important her blog was, how much comfort she took from readers' understanding.

---

87   John B. Dixon, MBBS, PhD, et al., "Adjustable Gastric Banding and Conventional Therapy for Type 2 Diabetes," *Journal of the American Medical Association* 299, no. 3 (January 23, 2008): 316–23.

88   Keith Taylor, ASMBS Fact Sheet, March 15, 2009, http://www.asmbs.org/Newsite07/media/asmbs_fs_surgery.pdf.

"People *get* what I'm talking about," she told Dr. Franks.

"What do you write about?" he asked.

"Stuff," she said. "My life."

"What stuff?"

"How I'm feeling at any given moment, what I find funny or offensive. Stuff."

"How are you feeling?" he asked.

She sighed. How many times did she have to tell him she lived in sadness the way a guppy lives in water, that she held a bowling ball of shame in her belly? "Okay," she answered.

"It sounds interesting, your blog."

"I'd really prefer you not read it. It's private."

"How can it be private if it's there for anyone to read?"

"It's my stuff. My readers share a lot of the same feelings. They write to tell me I'm okay."

"But anyone could read it and write to you that you're not okay. How would you feel about that?"

"Sad. But my friends would support me."

"Do you feel like I don't support you?"

What could she say? Dr. Franks was nice enough, but he was also one of the people who would be giving the go-ahead for her gastric bypass. And she wanted bypass more than anything in the world. She'd lost and gained 1,100 pounds in seventeen years. This third mountain of fat she had to pick her way down was too hard. She was profoundly, viscerally tired.

"Sure," she said. "I've been open with you, and I wouldn't have been if I didn't think you supported me. But I'd like you not to read my blog."

Dr. Frank read her blog. He read about her binges, her skirmishes with Kaiser over her gynecologist's rudeness, her sarcasm about the presurgery nutritionist who made her make a list of all the "illegal" foods she struggled with and then go out and buy them in specific quantities in some bizarre attempt to make friends with waffles. He read about how she wanted to kill herself on Christmas when her brothers ganged up on her for overreacting when her mother made a motel reservation for her rather than inviting her to stay in her old bedroom. He read about how she'd gotten two kittens despite her landlord's rules.

And then he told the committee that met to evaluate her candidacy that she wasn't ready, that she was immature, unable to stick to anything, given to wild mood swings, and unlikely to follow their medical, nutritional, and psychological advice.

"We feel you need more time," Laura, her nutritionist, called to tell her.

"Why?" Katie asked. "I've been through a year of meeting with you guys. I've jumped through all the hoops. What's the problem?"

"There are a number of problems, but mostly Dr. Franks is concerned about your suicidal tendencies. You barely survived Christmas, he says. He doesn't know how you'll handle your family as you're losing weight and they express their opinions about that."

Katie sat utterly still in her Barcalounger as Apple pulled at the fabric with her sharp claws, something that usually drove Katie nuts.

"Christmas?" she said in that whisper that would be a choke if she spoke any louder. "We didn't discuss Christmas."

"You must have or else—"

"He read my blog. He fucking read my blog. He fucking read my fucking blog after I fucking asked him not to. I can't believe this."

"Now, Katie—"

"Nuh-uh." Katie stopped her. "I've lived my whole fucking life with people like you saying 'Now, Katie' before they tell me I'm crazy or too emotional. He *read* my blog after I asked him not to. It's like he broke into my house and read my diaries! I can't believe this! There has to be some kind of law or rule or clause about prying." She started crying then. "And it doesn't matter, does it? Because all you guys have decided that because my family treated me like shit at Christmas and brought up old feelings of wanting to die, you'll let me commit suicide with food that you say I'm supposed to come to terms with. Because I got really sad, you're going to let me die, and they'll have to take my body out with a fucking crane!"

Laura listened, making occasional murmurs of understanding. At the end of the tirade, when Katie had given in to sobs, Laura cleared her throat and said, "We think it would be a good idea if you took my six-month class in mindful eating."

"I want a meeting with you, Dr. Franks. and Dr. Lefkowitz," Katie said, in that whisper that masks tears. "Kaiser's supposed to be a team. I want my team."

She got the meeting, but only after she'd slung every invective imaginable against her therapist and insurer on her blog. My personal favorite was calling Dr. Sneak an "ass-hat." Readers were sympathetic to her cry in the wilderness of fat—that she couldn't live this way anymore. They told her she had so much going for her, that fat or thin she was a wonderful person, that her shrink was a bastard.

I took a more nuts-and-bolts approach. "Get very calm. Make a list of how Kaiser has infringed upon your privacy. Explain how your blog reflects a bad day or a bad hour, not your general state of mind, and remind them of the statistics that show obese people are twenty-five percent more likely to be depressed. Also remind them of how many years of weighed-and-measured, restricted eating you've done, that you're perfectly capable of following a nutrition plan. Tell them how you're selling pet-sitting franchises and how well you're doing in a self-starter business, that you're a hard worker and show up for your life no matter how you're feeling. Go in there like a lawyer, not a beggar."

She thanked me for the advice although I don't know if or how capable she was of following it in her rage and, mostly, shame that she'd screwed up once again.

Compounding what had now become her notorious and permanent psychological profile, the surgeon stated that he was reluctant to put her on the operating table unless she lost weight.[89]

"Why?" she demanded. "I'm fat, but I don't have high blood pressure or diabetes. Lots of people who are fatter than I am have surgery."

"Anesthesia would be extremely risky," he said.

He tabled further discussion until she took Laura's class.

Mindful eating? we scoffed later. "I don't mind eating," she said.

"I don't mind it at all," I answered. "Would you mind passing the cake?"

"Sure, if you wouldn't mind ordering pizza."

Somehow, when disaster strikes Katie, it does so exponentially. Within a week of the Kaiser debacle, her landlord discovered Apple and Orange, and gave her two weeks to move out. It was lucky that the procedure had been put off.

"Who will rent to a four-hundred-poundy?" she wailed. "How can I possibly pack up my apartment when I can't stand for more than twenty minutes?"

Katie was due for a lesson in serendipity. She found a small apartment in Alamo that had a cocktail napkin–sized atrium. Her new proximity to Oakland revived old ideas of the way she wanted to live. College Avenue was Mecca for her, and the lights around Lake Merritt could keep a desperate woman hopeful. She decided Alamo was a step toward a bigger destiny. A few days later, when she placed

---

89 This was absurd. At five feet six inches and 419 pounds, Katie's body mass index was sixty-eight. The North American Association for the Study of Obesity advocates that bypass candidates have a minimum BMI of 40 or more without comorbid conditions, and 35 with one or more complications such as "cardiovascular, pulmonary, gastrointestinal, endocrine, and other obesity-related diseases." Edward Saltzman, et al., "Criteria for Patient Selection and Multidisciplinary Evaluation and Treatment of the Weight Loss Surgery Patient," *Obesity Research* 13 (2005), 234–43. Katie had not, however, stopped smoking, which is another prerequisite for weight-loss surgery. This was not brought up in her meeting.

an ad offering to give the rest of her thin clothes away so she wouldn't have to pack them, the respondent who swept up the pile of bags wept with gratitude because it would make her job search possible. In return, she recruited her brother and boyfriend with their trucks and they arrived on the Saturday of the move to do the whole job.

Could Katie have handled the gamut of weight-loss surgery? It is emphatically not for sissies, that's for damn sure.

A number of articulate and frank women responded to the note I put on the home page of my website asking for interviews with bariatric patients. One of them was Em. At five foot one, weighing 365 pounds, her life was on the line. Two years before having gastric bypass, she had her tonsils removed. The anesthesiologist arrived and gave her two injections in her neck, apologizing for the pain but explaining that it would take so much sodium pentothal to put her to sleep that he couldn't promise she'd wake up. She was awake for her tonsillectomy. Her evaluation for bypass surgery included an endoscopic examination of her upper gastrointestinal tract, and she was too heavy for sedation.

Sissies, indeed.

There are essentially three commonly used forms of weight-loss surgery that work through creating a small pouch at the top of the small intestine and bypassing the duodenum and upper portion of the jejunum where much of digestion takes place. The patient is restricted in the amount of food she can eat and cannot absorb many of the calories of the food she eats. These procedures are the vertical gastrectomy with duodenal switch (commonly referred to as the duodenal switch, or DS), the Roux-en-Y (the procedure referred to when using the phrase "gastric bypass" and often called RYGB—with about 140,000 such surgeries performed in the United States in 2005, it is the most popular form of WLS), and laparoscopic adjustable gastric banding (referred to as Lap-Banding).

An additional procedure, the vertical gastrectomy (known as VG), does not utilize malabsorption in weight loss. No portion of the intestines is bypassed but 90 percent of the small intestine is removed, reducing the amount the patient can initially eat to about two ounces, expanding as time goes on to about six ounces. There are only fifteen certified surgeons in the world performing this procedure.

All of this is big business. The cost of gastric bypass runs between eighteen and twenty-two thousand dollars for hospitalization, surgeon, and anesthesiologist's fees. Insurance companies are loath to hand out weight-loss surgeries but are persuadable if the surgeon documents the patient's medical need for it. Reconstructive surgery, nutrition counseling, and supplements,[90] psychotherapy, and exercise costs load on more expense, much of it not covered by insurers. A typical, high-end tummy tuck, for instance, can amount to more than fifteen thousand dollars, and may be combined with a body lift that ranges from twelve to fifty thousand. She may also need or want face (six to fifteen thousand) and breast lifts (three to six thousand), and liposuction.[91] An RYGB patient can spend up to sixty-six thousand dollars in surgical procedures when these fees are averaged. That's over nine million dollars a year in Roux-en-Y and skin reduction costs alone.

Bariatric surgery is a boomtown for surgeons, "the only general surgical procedure . . . for which practitioners actively advertise."[92] With stakes like that, the medical community promotes WLS as almost foolproof. It's not surprising, then, that finding hard data on the risks of surgery is not an easy task.

---

90   The bypassed duodenum and jejunum results in lack of iron, calcium, and B-12 absorption. Some surgeries also require supplements of vitamins A, D, E, and K.

91   Neil Hutcher, MD, "Cost of Weight Loss (Bariatric) Surgery," April 20, 2009, http://www.yourplasticsurgeryguide.com/bariatric/cost.htm (accessed).

92   J. Eric Oliver, *Fat Politics* (New York: Oxford University Press, 2006), 54.

One such study was conducted by a team from the University of Massachusetts Medical School on a pool of 188 RYGB patients. In the year following their surgeries, fifty of them had complications severe enough that a second surgery was required. Two patients died. The study concluded that sleep apnea, hypertension, and surgical inexperience were predictors of future complications.[93]

There is also ample evidence of nutritionally compromised spinal cords, peripheral nerve damage, and brain complications that can set in from two weeks to several years after surgery. These neurologic complications seem to result from the lack of thiamine, copper, and vitamin B12 absorption from food.[94] Complications, running from leaks to hernias, various infections, and increased chances of developing kidney stones, add yet more expense.

For all surgeries, weight loss peaks at twelve to eighteen months, at which time there is usually a ten- to fifteen-pound weight gain because that palm-sized pouch has stretched to the size of two cupped hands. A significant portion of WLS patients manage to stretch their pouch, despite dumping,[95] enough that as many as 10 percent of WLS patients return to their original weight after two years, and almost 30 percent of some WLS procedures produce no maintained weight loss at all.[96] Gina Kolata notes that despite large losses, most patients remain above the demarcation line of obesity, a BMI of 30.[97]

---

93   Richard A. Perugini, et al., "Predictors of Complications and Suboptimal Weight Loss After Laparascopic Roux-en-Y Gastric Bypass: a Series of 188 Patients," *Archives of Surgery* (May 2003): 541–46.

94   K. Juhasz-Poscine, S. A. Rudnicki, R. L. Archer, S. I. Harik, "Neurologic Complications of Gastric Bypass Surgery for Morbid Obesity," *Neurology* 68 (2007): 1843–50.

95   "Dumping" refers to any combination of the following: sweating, weakness, bloating, faintness, and/or cramping. It occurs when undigested food is released too quickly into the small intestine.

96   Oliver, 55.

97   Gina Kolata, *Rethinking Thin* (New York: Farrar Straus & Giroux, 2007), 58.

Part of insurers' criteria for the surgery is proof that no other weight management program will work for the individual. All WLS patients are many-times-over failures before they meet their anesthesiologist. The women I spoke to for this book take their past failures as serious warnings of what could begin at any moment, and all of them have witnessed failures from their surgical groups. Even with weight-loss surgery, they worry that they'll fail. Bariatric surgery is no guarantee of permanent weight loss. I met two women, Cynthia and Karen, for whom their Lap-Bands ultimately failed.

The introductory literature WLS candidates receive must state that the contemplated procedure is a tool, not a cure, because Karen, Cynthia, and Katie have all used the phrase.

Seven years ago, at the age of twenty-four, Karen dropped a hundred pounds to 145 on a low-carbohydrate diet. The change was so dramatic that her law school classmates thought she was a transfer student when she returned for their second year. A terrible first boss sent her back to chocolate, and her weight skyrocketed to 274 pounds. Karen met her husband at 145 pounds and he proposed to her 130 pounds later but she worried that he loved her *despite* her weight.

That was why she decided to have surgery, and she has regretted it ever since. After Lap-Band, she's gone from 274 (BMI 44) pounds to 171 (BMI 27.4) then up to 230 and down to 170. With the band too tight for the salads and proteins she considered proper weight-loss food, she woke up choking with reflux in the middle of the night and had stuck to "squishy" foods since. In her third upswing in as many years, she weighed 224 pounds. "I wasn't aware of the complications of eating," she said. Karen eventually joined Overeaters Anonymous, giving up sugar and white flour. Her Lap-Band slipped and she had to have it removed.

"People can use [the surgery] and lose weight or go back to their old lifestyle and try later," Cynthia observed. She knows this from her own experience.

Failure is easy with the move, after a couple of weeks, from protein shakes to soft foods such as milk shakes or mashed potatoes and gravy. Because of the interim soft-food diet, Cynthia didn't change the method of how she ate. The move to whole food, which she wolfed in her customary manner, made her violently ill. "I'd be out at a restaurant and have two or three bites, get up, and vomit. Mom called the band my choke chain around my stomach. If it was liquid, I could eat a gallon, but after a bite or two of substance, I was done. And it would hurt." And so she ate the gallon of liquid, and her initial weight of 280 pounds dropped to 230 in the first six postoperative months and stayed there.

Frustrated with her Lap-Band failure, a year and a half later, she underwent vertical gastrectomy and had 90 percent of her stomach removed, including the portion that produces gherlin, one of the hormones that tells the brain we're hungry. (This is perhaps the only aspect of any of the surgeries I personally envy. Oh, to be released from hunger!) Unlike the other surgeries, the VG doesn't rearrange the stomach, so there is less propensity to dumping and nausea. This aspect of the surgery, Cynthia said, "puts the responsibility squarely on the patient's shoulders. Your body isn't going to punish you for what or the way you eat." In the eighteen months since the surgery, she has dropped from 230 to 140 pounds and is working toward a goal of 125 pounds.

The costs are enormous. Cynthia had two surgeries and body-lift surgery,[98] which she wanted in order to better unite the thin girl walking down the street with the girl on the beach or in the bedroom.

---

98   The folds of skin left after dramatic weight loss are breeding grounds for bacterial and fungal infections and they can be as uncomfortable as the fat was before because of rubbing and girdling. On the other hand, contouring plastic surgery is more invasive than the original bariatric procedure, with fluid and blood collections at the extensive wound site (the resulting scars can run twelve inches), possibly more blood loss, as well as a much longer and more bedridden recovery time. The surgeries—belly, thighs, arms, breast, and face—are not usually performed in one procedure because of the dangers of lengthy anesthesia. Ranit Mishori, "Leaving the Folds: After a Gastric Bypass, Some Formerly Obese Patients Need a Riskier Surgery to Shed Excess Skin," *Washington Post*, May 30, 2006.

No matter how great she looked clothed, the apron of excess skin on her stomach and sagging breasts made her reluctant to show herself beyond a certain stage of undress. Her marriage was also part of the price of the surgeries. "My husband married a morbidly obese girl, and that's what made sense in his world." Add in the cost of a divorce.

Vertical gastrectomy sounds infallible, but it's had its failures. Worried after her failure with her Lap-Band, Cynthia asked her doctor if anyone ever bombed out on the new procedure. He told her he'd had two patients who never lost a pound. "It is possible to sabotage any surgery if you are determined, I guess," she said ruefully.

But there are far more success stories than failures. Betsy's bottom came when she could no longer look at herself in the mirror, even from the neck up. "I was so unhealthy, on so many medications for high blood pressure and high cholesterol. I couldn't get out of bed in the morning. I hated life, hated myself. I couldn't white-knuckle through Weight Watchers one more time. Surgery was my last chance in life." The cost for her was mortgaging her house when, as a single parent, she had two kids in college.

The mortgage was her weapon in making her Lap-Band surgery work. "I went in with the attitude that it was sixteen thousand dollars out of my pocket—I make a penny scream, I pinch it so hard. Maybe people who don't have to mortgage their house don't have to commit to the process."

Lap-Band is the least invasive procedure, but it often requires several follow-ups to get the right "fit" of the Silastic Ring around the newly created stomach pouch. Betsy had three saline "fills" through the port to get the correct feeling of restriction.

One of the ironies of most of the weight-loss surgeries is that what we think of as "diet" food is nearly impossible to eat. Raw vegetables, salads, dense proteins such as meat, sugar-free soda, and caffeine all cause a suffocating panic from the food getting stuck. Betsy said she either vomited or the food would eventually go down, but the experience was terrifying.

One of the reasons that Em, Karen, Cynthia, and Betsy were willing to discuss the reality of their experiences is that it was, simply, a chance to talk. Most bariatric surgery centers have patient groups, but they were, according to Betsy and Cynthia, so full of newbies that it was tough to talk about raw versus baked apples or being with a new friend who made a nasty comment about a fatso walking down the street.

Nor did they have comrades to talk with about how the habit of reaching for food as comfort didn't leave. "The physical procedure was easiest," Betsy said. "I never ate for hunger anyway. It was 'I'm bored, I'm happy, I'm depressed, there goes a yellow VW.' The day you say, 'Oh, screw it, I'll eat a box of Ding-Dongs,' you can only have three because you don't have a stomach. Unfortunately, they don't put a band on your head."

"I'm scared of that point where I'm not losing weight anymore," Cynthia confessed of the fifteen to twenty pounds her doctor feels she can, if she wants, still lose. "Do I ever get to live a normal life where I don't worry about what I get to eat or how much I exercise? My brother had vertical gastric in June and is down to 190, which is a healthy weight for him, and we were joking that I had ninety percent of my stomach removed and now I need part of my head removed. My brain still says, 'you're fat, you're angry.' What do I do with that?"

I've always said I'd consider weight-loss surgery if it came with a lobotomy.

Such a bargain is not so far off the mark. When a woman decides to have gastric surgery, she must, in order to be successful, change her relationship with the how and the why of her eating. There are really only three relationships one can have with the staff of life: the lucky few who eat for fuel, the extremely unlucky who eat for the sake of eating, and the mixed blessing of eating for the luxurious sake of the food itself.

A woman who has gotten to the size that she needs surgery to reverse it probably eats as a way of living. The food she ate in the past was important mainly for satisfying either an emotional need or a need beyond need, an imperative to chew, fill up, medicate. The hardcore eater, like Cynthia, doesn't take small bites and chew carefully: she *feeds*. After surgery, the patient has to learn to eat, mindfully, for nutrition. If she wants a sensuous relationship with food, it will be in bits and drabs, and in the surprises of new foods she is allowed to eat.

The Angry Fat Girls and other relapsers must take these classifications as seriously as the surgical patient. Answering this question is a purely individual but fraught product of a lot of reflection—and it's essential. Do we eat to eat, or do we have a different kind of relationship with food?

Mimi, for one, wanted eat her cake and savor it, too. She loved food. She loved the sensation of gelato in her mouth, was a student of pad thai, swooned over her Rachel Ray fruitcake. She had an educated palate and noticed things like the taste of wax in See's chocolates or the use of powdered garlic instead of fresh. She even made a point of not eating everything on her plate . . . only to trip up soon after. "I made the mistake of eating a gingersnap after breakfast," she berated herself on her personal blog. "The taste was addictive to the point that I brought the rest of the bag with me and ate in the car as I drove."

I think the Skinny Cow chocolate peanut butter ice cream sandwich is a trick to make us think we can have it both ways. "Of course you can have it all," its website proclaims under the banner of "Livin' Large by Livin' Skinny." Tossing phrases and words like "rich and creamy deliciousness," "creamy, dreamy, guilt-free," and "give in to temptation" around like confetti, the peppy cow doesn't really make a case for moderation or, better yet, learning to control cravings. "Some open their minds. Others open their hearts. Me, I open my freezer," says the website's cow with "sass." We're suckered in because the unspoken promise in Right Bites is that all we have to do is lose weight and then we can have more.

So, no, Wendy's fat-free refried beans do not count as a vegetable and aren't a substitute for broccoli. Such self-delusions don't pay off. They don't realign our use of food, the how and the why. Nor does a 140-calorie ice cream bar fill the void that the big bag of potato chips did.

Successful dieting is forever. If we maintain our weight loss, we never leave the diet, so the bargain we have to strike is between starving because our weekly points are used up or using those weekly points to put true, physical hunger to rest. For many women, I suspect, food is a lot like marriage and may even be the secret lover in many actual marriages. In our union with pizza, we have a choice between constant arguing and pretending the relationship is healthy, or our wedlock falls somewhere on the continuum between marriage counseling and divorce. Gastric bypass is a divorce. The torturous daily assessment of food as "good" or "bad" is having a misogamist for a shrink. The rigid food plan that Karen now follows is a legal separation with the intent to divorce sometime before she dies. "OA has been difficult," she wrote me, "but [it] has also given me a freedom I have not experienced in a long time."

Extreme measures leave us in a lifelong moment of truth about what food means to us, what its absence means to us, and how we must craft a sense of self apart from all its charms and consequences. Surviving food's absence and exploring ourselves is part of what happened when Wendy asked if we could start a joint blog. Blogging for Angry Fat Girlz meant a certain amount of meditation and research, and it required the focus that a package of Vienna Fingers once got. The responses were a wedge in our loneliness. For an hour or so every other day, either on Angry Fat Girlz or our own blogs, we were free of eating and in the thrall of our own talents and intelligence.

We were ourselves.

ELEVEN

February

"You Are My Candy Girl"

The deliverymen watched Katie lie down on her new bed. She refused to imagine what they were thinking, this refrigerator of a woman whomping down on the plastic-covered mattress and box springs that sang a couple of bars of a nursery rhyme until her four hundred pounds settled. The box springs toottled again—was it "Peter, Peter, pumpkin-eater"?—as she pushed hard with her left forearm to roll over onto her right side. She raised her right arm and rested her head on it.

"No," she said, with her back to the two guys. They were kind of dishy, absolutely the sort of men she feared most, the ones who'd write "No fat girls need apply" in a personal ad, or might, on a horny Friday night, go on Craigslist hunting for big game they could do the nasty with and then disappear into tall tales at their favorite sports bar. "It's not right. It's not the one I tried at the store."

"It's the same model numbers," one of them said, and rattled off some gibberish that ended in "extra firm."

"I don't care. It's not right. I want the one from the showroom."

"We delivered the same units, ma'am, but we didn't pick up no showroom mattresses."

"Then call and tell them you're returning these and pick up the showroom mattress and box springs that I tried out."

"We can take these back," the other one said, "but you'll have to call about the showroom model and make new arrangements for delivery."

Katie rolled off to the edge of the bed, swung her feet to the floor, and leveraged herself over so that she could stand by pushing up from the mattress with her hands. She faced them and said, "No. Call right now and tell them you're making the switch."

"We told you, ma'am, we just pick up from the warehouse. We don't work for the showroom."

"Well, you do now," she snapped. "Take these out and bring back the showroom models."

"'Ma'am' got a little snippy today," Katie told me on the phone that night. She was snuggled in her new showroom-floor double bed, leaning up against a reading bolster, her old yellow quilt pulled up to her chin. Orange was settled at her feet, and Apple was curled just under the bolster. "I made them take the mattresses back and deliver what I wanted in the same afternoon. I ended up calling the manager and told him I was too sleepy not to get what I paid for on the day it was promised."

"I'm impressed." And I was. We obese women overtip, get pressured into buying more expensive cell phones and laptops, all the while that we are fawningly thanking clerks and telling stores it's not a problem that it will take another week for delivery. We do this as an act of begging pardon for taking up so much space, for stepping out of the invisibility of being fat by asking for things.

"Me, too. But, Frances—I'm in bed!"

Her old bed, thrown out in the move, had been intolerable for the last couple of years, and she'd been sleeping in the La-Z-Boy recliner she had to replace at least once a year. The feel of sheets on her bare legs was heaven.

"You know what else?" she asked. Katie is the most excitable of us, not only prone to despair but also to the thrill of treats. She has never waited to open a Christmas or birthday present in her life. "I haven't done much grocery shopping yet. The only stuff in my kitchen is Diet Coke, skim milk, lettuce, tomatoes, and a cooked chicken breast. And apples. And olive oil and vinegar that made the move."

"Are you going to get some vegetables and breakfast stuff today?"

"Mmm," she said noncommittally. "The thing is, this is the first abstinent kitchen I've ever had. So far. It's been a week and I've binged, but not at home."

"Wow." I know what it's like to throw out flour and sugar, honey and bread, working my way down to alcohol-based extracts and, eventually, the rolling pin and cake pans. "Are you planning to stay in bed in order to keep it that way?"

"No. I'm planning on going to a meeting in Oakland tonight. There's a huge one at a hospital at seven. Much as I hate the thought of going to another damn hospital."

The meeting was held in a small auditorium. Katie wasn't sure which was worse, the twenty or so people already there or the auditorium chairs. She was grateful, and a little furious, when someone noticed her hesitation and got up and set out a couple of folding chairs in the front row.

Right where the worst fatties could be inspected and pitied. Poor things: I hope the Higher Power doesn't let that happen to me . . .

To her relief, other people drifted in and hauled over more folding chairs. By the time the leader stepped up to the podium and invited the crowd to stand and join the Serenity Prayer, there were a dozen women sitting in the row with Katie.

The meeting started with a reading of the twelve steps and a new arrival took the seat that would be least disruptive of the proceedings. That chair was next to Katie. She shifted her bulk to the left as much as she could without entering her other neighbor's space and concentrated on what was being read.

"Number Three," a man's voice from the back announced. "Made a decision to turn our will and our lives to the care of God as we understood him."

"Number Four," another man's voice picked up. "Made a searching and fearless inventory of ourselves."

Katie groaned inwardly. She's been in the Rooms for fifteen years and had worked the steps. They had not prevented her from getting to 427 pounds. Other people seemed to be able to practice all those twelve-steppy niblets of advice—keep your eyes on your own plate; one day at a time; let go, let God—but they seemed to have some extra epidermis or a curtain they could pull to keep the world in its place. Katie felt like a burn victim, missing her skin, or like she lived behind a scrim where her reactions and desires were on freak show display.

The leader introduced a speaker named Kenneth. Katie slumped. Men's and women's experiences with eating, food, weight, body image, the program, life were so different that it could void the story's validity for the opposite sex.

He talked about growing up in chaos, a rageful alcoholic father, a meek mother who didn't defend herself or her six kids. Early on, he discovered he felt safe when he was stuffed. Sometimes he ate plain flour to achieve what he had come to understand was the indifference of numbness. He weighed three hundred pounds when he barely managed to graduate from high school. Getting a job at Wal-Mart got him out of his parents' house, and it got him easy access to candy bars, bags of cookies, stale bakery goods on sale.

He ballooned to four hundred pounds in a year and got fired for shoplifting a fistful of Snickers bars. He spent his unemployment in his room, watching television and eating. When his unemployment ran out, he got a night job as a janitor in a hospital where he mostly hung out in waiting rooms. That's where he heard about Optifast and dropped 220 pounds in a year. He enrolled in night school and studied computer science. He got buff. He got his first boyfriend. They started eating out, and he learned he was a talented cook. They had regular Sunday brunches. His weight shot up. His boyfriend dumped him.

By then he was working in information technology for the hospital and heard about something else, a twelve-step program for compulsive eating. He gave it a shot.

"I can't tell you that my life is easy," he said. "My father died of ammonia on the brain last year, and my mother had a nervous breakdown. As the only sibling who doesn't have kids, I was the one who had to check her into a hospital and look after her when she came home. It meant moving back to the place where my disease took away my life. But I did it abstinently. I didn't eat sugar or flour, I measured my meals, I continued to pray and meditate. Sometimes I stood at the kitchen cupboards looking at what was in them. But my sponsor reminded me that God loves me as I am, but He loves me too much to keep where I am. I knew it was only temporary and mostly I did what they say in OA—don't eat, read the Big Book, go to meetings. Because I'd made my amends to my parents and let go of a lot of my bitterness toward them, I was able to finally see that serenity is not freedom from the storm but peace amid the storm."

The timekeeper was holding her hands up in a T to signify that his time was up. He nodded and smiled—at Katie, especially?—and said, "I'll just close by saying, keep coming back!"

The applause was thunderous. Everybody loves a huge weight-loss success. Katie clapped, too. That thing about God loving a person too much to keep them where they are hit close to her new home. She'd been kicked out of her San Bruno apartment because of the kittens she loved. Her dream of gastric bypass was busted. She was in that

storm that Kenneth talked about, a storm of rejection, but she had
no serenity. It was another aphorism that works for people who can
pull down heavy drapes and secede from other people's bad weather.
When Katie tried to shut out bullshit like Kaiser's evaluation team
and her mother's assumption that she'd take the cats to the ASPCA
and apologize to her old landlord, her scrim was too flimsy to hold out
against a rain-lashed wind.

Katie felt a hand on her knee. It was the woman at her right, the
one who came in during the steps. Diane! Diane, her first sponsor
from seventeen years ago!

"Oh, my God!" Katie squealed. A couple of disapproving looks
shot their way, and she lowered her voice. "How are you?"

"I'm good, Katie. How are you?" Diane's whisper was tentative.
She could see perfectly well how Katie was. Stevie Wonder could see
how Katie was doing.

She opened her hands. *Duh.* "Let's talk after the meeting," Diane
said, and sat back with her legs crossed, holding Katie's hand for the
next forty minutes. The warmth of Diane's hand and the steady pressure as she gently squeezed Katie's knuckles allowed her to cry.

"I had a sponsor last spring who put me on the Kay Sheppard
plan," Katie told Diane over coffee. "I lost a little weight but it was
slow and the plan is stupid."

Diane is a small woman with bright blue eyes. She was a little
plumper than the last time Katie saw her, some ten years ago or so,
and she'd let her hair go gray. Her curls bobbed as she nodded her
head.

"Stupid how?"

Katie ticked off the forbidden substances: "No caffeine. No diet
soda. No aspartame, NutraSweet, or Splenda: only saccharine or ste-
via. Sugar-free toothpaste at seven bucks a tube. One teaspoon of
spice or herbs a day. One ounce of vinegar or salsa or mustard or other
condiment per day. I mean, what the fuck?"

"But you were losing weight?"

"Like, thirty pounds in two months. I know, I know. Lots of people would be thrilled to lose twenty pounds. Lots of people don't weigh more than four hundred pounds and aren't on disability and trying to qualify for weight-loss surgery. But my sponsor decided that at my weight, I should eat the men's version of the food plan. Six ounces of protein and six ounces of dairy for breakfast, a starch at every meal. A protein and fruit 'metabolic adjustment.' I was always eating, and it was too much food."

"Does this plan associate itself with Program?" Diane asked.

"Yeah. I was going to meetings and studying the Big Book with my sponsor. I didn't like her, though. I mean, I liked her, but I hated going over to her house."

Diane shook her head. She'd heard Katie's screwball reasoning before. Thirteen years earlier, Katie raved in her morning phone calls about how much she loved her new boss at the Department of Justice; she was high on the mob case he was pursuing, her coworkers were hilarious . . . but the office was painted a bilious green that ground her nerves. Then there was the new best friend from the Rooms. They shopped for their new thin clothes together, went to the movies, went hiking in Muir Woods. But the young woman didn't have an answering machine and that was, in a daily gathering of grievances, the end of that.

Diane knew these enthusiasms were surrogates for food. Katie didn't fall out of love with people or interests or work as much as she hurtled through them, ravenously, until she came abruptly to some aspect of herself that she despised. It wasn't the paint, it was the feeling that she was helping to put crooks away when what she really wanted to do was de-crook them. Her answering machineless friend was her lifeline, and Katie hated herself for needing a savior. The damage she did was through her inability to let a friendship wane or leave a job gracefully. She would quit without explanations or apologies, not because she hated who or what she was leaving but because she hated herself for her hunger.

Katie had quit Diane. A friend from the Rooms had migrated to a cousin program and Katie followed. Diane didn't see her in meetings or hear from her for a couple of weeks. She called and left a message, and Katie responded by email that she'd started going to FA.

Looking at her now, Diane was impressed that Katie had returned to the Rooms. It spoke volumes about the power of the basic premises of community and repetition one finds there.

"It sounds like this—Kay Sheppard?—wasn't the food plan for you," Diane said cautiously. "What are you eating now?"

"Pretty much everything, but not at home. At home I eat abstinently. Mostly I don't eat there."

Diane laughed. "I've always thought car insurance should be higher for active food addicts. Eating a hero and driving Nimitz Freeway is a menace to society."

"Dipping french fries in those little ketchup things during rush hour on Van Ness should be short-listed as an Olympic event. And I drive a stick shift."

"The things we do for our disease." Diane took a long sip of her coffee. "So I take it you don't have a sponsor."

"No. I just moved here. This is my first meeting in—phoo. Months."

"You've moved to Oakland?"

"No. Alamo. Or Vanillaville, whichever. It's the world's most boring town."

"Do you want to get abstinent?"

Katie's eyes teared up at that. She looked quickly down at her coffee cup and stirred it diligently. "More than anything," she said hoarsely.

"What kind of abstinence are you looking for? You've certainly sampled a bunch."

"I want the basics. The way I did it with you. Three meals, low carbohydrate, no seven-dollar toothpaste or being forbidden to eat out for the first ninety days."

"Do you want a sponsor?"

"Are you offering to sponsor me?"

"Yes."

Diane handed a wad of napkins to Katie, which she blindly reached for, and held her hand tightly as Katie cried.

It is one of the most magical moments in life, when desperation tunnels through one's soul and emerges into the light of courage and one is able to ask someone for help with food, the most intimate, meaningful object in life. Consider that Katie weighed 411 pounds that day and was barely able to go to the supermarket. She thought that she was a monster, whom no one would sit next to or touch on purpose, that she had been put on display in the meeting. A month earlier, she was convinced no one would rent an apartment to her, or that her boss would fire her when she went to the first sales meeting and he saw what she looked like. Her family had done everything it could to let her know how unwelcome she was in their midst, and her therapist had betrayed her best shot at losing weight.

And there she was, in a pink hospital coffee shop being offered a second chance by a woman who knew she was wildly emotional, unpredictable, a failure at everything. Jesus, she'd failed Diane, and she was offering her time and hope anyway.

In turn, Katie would write down each day's food and call it in to Diane every morning. She would report any deviations from the day's menu. She would tell her when things were horrible and when things were good, and Diane would cajole her to go to a meeting either way and to not eat over it.

Even if Katie had serious doubts about Program, after failing at it so many times in so many ways, it was the only thing she'd ever done that worked.

After her talk with Diane, Katie had her last night of drive-ins. At McDonald's, she flicked open her cell phone and consulted an imaginary lover about what he wanted before ordering two large orders of fries with four packs of ketchup and a large chocolate shake. She ate that star combo of hot and cold, crispy and soft, salty and sweet, in the parking lot of the Safeway next door, consuming 2,200 calories of bliss. Then she drove to Popeye's for a sort of normal dinner of chicken, biscuits, mashed potatoes and gravy, which she ate in the franchise's parking lot. Katie would join me in saying "sort of" because we both know that the nutrition in her chicken was massively overbalanced by fat. She would not be surprised to know that the stop cost her not only seven bucks but 1,500 calories, which is more than either of us eats in a day when we are losing weight on our food plans.

Her final stop was Dairy Queen, where she she waited while a guy on his cell phone dithered about what he wanted. She ended up ordering two large Blizzards, an Oreo and a Snicker at 980 and 1,140 calories respectively.

Her drive home from Oakland was a last hurrah of 5,820 calories while maintaining a kitchen that would be used for abstinent cooking the next morning.

This is beyond the "mindless eating"[99] that Brian Wansink blames the statistics of obesity on, or Geneen Roth's "emotional eating,"[100] which is a substitute reaction to feelings, although both authors make salient points about America's expanding waistlines. This was a last embrace of a lover that gripped her as tangibly as the lover on her cell phone was a fake.

The eighteen months of writing *Eating Ice Cream with My Dog* were punctuated by a number of books that took a second, closer look at the obesity epidemic and diet industry. With hard science to back them up, J. Eric Oliver, Brian Wansink, Gina Kolata, Gary Taubes, and David S.

---

99   Brian Wansink, *Mindless Eating: Why We Eat More Than We Think* (New York: Bantam Books, 2006).

100   See any one of Geneen Roth's many books on the subject: *Breaking Free from Emotional Eating* (New York: Plume, 2003); *Feeding the Hungry Heart: The Experience of Emotional Eating* (New York: Macmillan, 1992); *When Food Is Love: Exploring the Relationship Between Eating and Intimacy* (New York: Dutton, 1991).

Kessler scrutinize what and how we eat and, in the cases of Oliver and Kolata, the improbability that we can or even should lose weight.[101] And yet, for as much information as Oliver and Kolata give about how the roles of genetics and hormones predetermine an individual's weight, they do not consider how other biological scripts make us fat. Let's face it: it's really hard to get fat from eating too much steamed cauliflower. Those calories have to be coming, in consistent and big quantities, from somewhere else. And they have to be doing something besides filling up our stomachs on the way home from an emotionally charged OA meeting with abstinence on the stroke of midnight.

Those calories make us feel, temporarily, better, and one of the messengers in the brain that is increased by high blood sugar is serotonin, the neurotransmitter that regulates body temperature, alertness and sleep, concentration, memory, creativity, and emotion.

I look at those by-products of serotonin and think they sound great. Who wouldn't want more creativity or serotonin's enhancement of memory?

The problem, according to Joan Ifland, in conjunction with Gilbert Manso, MD, is that the tide of serotonin flooding the brain makes us drunk. "Serotonin alone will make us feel confused, dazed, foggy, and sleepy."[102]

What did Katie do as soon as she got home? She flopped into that new bed of hers and zoned out on *Saturday Night Live*, which she loved but was too full to laugh at.

---

101   J. Eric Oliver, *Fat Politics*; Brian Wansink, *Mindless*; Gina Kolata, *Rethinking Thin* (New York: Farrar Straus & Giroux, 2007); Gary Taubes, *Good Calories, Bad Calories: Challenging the Conventional Wisdom on Diet, Weight Control, and Disease* (New York: Alfred A. Knopf, 2007); David S. Kessler, *The End of Overeating: Taking Control of the Insatiable American Appetite* (New York: Rodale, 2009).

102   Joan Ifland, *Sugars and Flours: How They Make Us Crazy, Sick, and Fat and What to Do about It* (Bloomington, IN: 1st Books Library, 2003), 28.

Elevated blood sugar also stimulates the manufacture of endorphins, or opioids, which affect the reward-and-pleasure center of the brain. This sense of reward is activated by the sensations of food and is so involuntary that we react to even the expectation of food. I see this every day with my dog, who licks her lips whenever she does something "good" (peeing or taking a dump, not lunging at a dog or person she dislikes) outside and on leash. Like the opiates (codeine, morphine, heroin) they resemble, writes David A. Kessler:

> the opioids produced by eating high-sugar, high-fat foods can relieve pain or stress and calm us down. At least in the short run, they make us feel better—we see this in infants who cry less when given sugar water. We can also observe that animals feel less pain when they're administered opioid-like drugs and even less [pain] when they're allowed unrestricted access to sucrose at the same time.[103]

Completing the sugar-charged triumvirate of brain chemicals is dopamine, the neurotransmitter that affects motivation, cognition, and voluntary movement, all of which prodded Katie to plot her drive home from Oakland in order to get her rewards at her favorite spots and be able to eat in the peace and privacy she prefers. Dopamine gives the oomph to do the work that a reward requires.

While likening some people's desire for particular foods to the desire alcoholics have to drink, shoplifters have to steal, and compulsive gamblers to pull up a chair at a roulette table, Kessler considers "hyperpalliative" (i.e., easy to eat and really yummy) foods habit-forming rather than addicting. He mentions Alcoholics Anonymous and Al-Anon as models for how to stop their particular behaviors but he never mentions twelve-step help for bad eaters. At least by

---

103   Kessler, 37–38.

ignoring it, he doesn't misunderstand it.[104] Instead, Kessler devises a vague cognitive approach to weight loss: if only Katie had deliberately taken a different route home, using residential streets rather than the fast-food strips, if only she had committed to having grilled chicken and salad that night, if only she had coached herself in how awful she would feel in the morning, she could have avoided ingesting more than five thousand calories and the cravings she had the next day when she told Diane she would have four ounces of chicken at dinner.

But could Katie have reasoned herself out of what Kessler calls the "cue-urge-reward-habit" cycle?

Katie and I, like millions of other people, consider ourselves addicted to sugar, wheat, and refined carbohydrates. They are mood-altering substances that replace the world of negative emotions we live in. What was really going on as she lay on her bed and watched *SNL*? Katie, at 411 pounds, took up no space at all, so snugly wrapped in that sunken, inert, carefree, Teflon-coated space that was big enough only for her and a remote control. An expert in manipulating foods, she had fed perfectly in order to gain that state. "Guess what food combines tryptophan [the precursor of serotonin] and sweets?" Anne Katherine posits. "Ice cream, a staple for most overeaters."[105]

No shit.

Katie woke at seven in order to call Diane, and while she felt great hope and relief—"the pink cloud" of twelve-step programs—her voice was thick with her hangover's need for more sleep. She hauled herself

---

104   Indeed, J. Eric Oliver, who improperly hyphenates *overeaters*, uses it as part of a cultural wave: "the emaciated Twiggy emerged as a beauty icon, when anorexia nervosa became a widespread disorder, when diet organizations such as Weight Watchers and Over-Eaters [sic] Anonymous were founded, when diet books became best sellers ..." *Fat Politics*, 85. Gina Kolata discusses OA in the same paragraph as TOPS and caricatures it by tying it to Hollywood and its spiritual ties to AA. *Rethinking Thin*, 58.

105   Anne Katherine, MA, *Anatomy of a Food Addiction: The Brain Chemistry of Overrating* (Corlobod, CA: Gürze Books, 1991), 39.

to the kitchen and drank two big glasses of water, took a Diet Coke from the fridge, and went back to bed. The aftermath of such a night wasn't any prettier than the garbage she'd thrown out at a 7-Eleven on the way home. She stayed in bed that day and watched a season's worth of *Project Runway*, barely managing to make a breakfast of a banana and yogurt after one in the afternoon. Thanking God it was Sunday, she had no energy, no mood at all, no motivation, no expectations. The day had only one challenge: three weighed and measured meals, no sugar, no flour.

On Tuesday, she emailed me that, "The most amazing feeling came over me as I ate that first abstinent meal. I felt like I was 'home.' I hadn't had that feeling is so long. It feels solid, secure, free. I have freedom. I feel less scared, less depressed, touched by God. I haven't felt touched by God in three years. I'm weeping as I write this out of gratitude. I can't believe how glad I am that my food is simplified. I'm free of searching for all these ways to control my eating. I don't have to think, which is good . . ." She was parched for more of the self-esteem she was amassing, but as Sheppard and Katherine warn, the succeeding days found her fretting over what she had done to herself in the last two years, raging at a godless universe when she was supposed to be saying the Serenity Prayer, looking for a hit of something—a new Must-See TV show or alphabetizing her books—to take the edge off the boredom of not eating through the days, her fear and frustration around her life, and the damp February chill of northern California.

Those are the dangerous days, the last seven of the first ten. The relief tapers off as the body detoxes without a brain that has been trained to supply the serotonin/endorphins/dopamine only when it is turned on by sugar. Katie's nerves felt like they had been run over by a cheese grater, and she had the shakes, diarrhea, a compelling thirst that couldn't be bought off, and crying jags. Diane advised her to drink lots of water and to get as much sleep as possible—and make calls to people in Program, go to meetings, read her daily meditation book, and pray, pray, pray.

I didn't hear from Katie for a couple of weeks after that and I understood why. Early abstinence is a silent, selfish time. Finding the words for email is difficult, and my abstinence was also so shaky that Katie really couldn't risk a phone conversation. I was viral and I knew it. She had her eyes glued to her own feet as she lifted out of the detox and started to fight for a future that would unfold as slowly as she lost weight.

Katie—and I—are perfectly normal in our responses to sugar. Sugar (and sugars derived from refined carbohydrates), science is starting to show us, replaces or enhances the felicitous hormones and neurotransmitters so effectively that an alteration in the brain's neural synapses occurs.

At the 2005 convention of the Western Psychological Association, Bartley Hoebel, PhD, presented his findings on experiments with rats allowed unlimited access to sugar. After ten days, they were given naloxone, a drug that blocks many of the brain's neurotransmitters and external opiates.

The rats showed some of the same withdrawal symptoms, such as teeth chattering and forepaw tremors, that mark withdrawal from an addictive drug. The naloxone-treated rats also showed decreased levels of dopamine and increased levels of acetylcholine [a neurotransmitter that, among other things, rouses excitement, arousal, and reward] in the brain—another sign of withdrawal.[106]

Sugar is as much a drug, Hoebel concluded, as heroin or cocaine—and it works on exactly the same center of the brain that heroin does. "There is something about this combination of heightened opioid and

---

106   Lea Winerman, "Intelligence, Sugar and the Cat-lot Hustle Headline WPA Meeting," *American Psychological Association Monitor on Psychology* 36, no. 6 (June 2005): 38.

dopamine responses in the brain that leads to dependency," explains Hoebel. "Without these neurotransmitters, the animal begins to feel anxious and wants to eat sweet food again."[107] And like other addictions, "users keep seeking."

Is it any wonder that the writers of the Big Book of Alcoholics Anonymous recommend that recovering alcoholics have chocolate and sweets constantly at hand?[108] Is it any wonder I laugh derisively whenever I see a commercial selling rum that pairs the liquor with diet cola and announces "zero sugar"? Why doesn't the nutrition, diet, and neuroscience literature more closely compare an intolerance for alcohol with an intolerance for sugar?

The worst of this self-produced and willfully amped pharmacopoeia isn't over yet. It gets worse because it can change the brain. By overwhelming the brain with glucose-induced opioids and mood-enhancing hormones, receptors begin to shut down and more external stimulation is needed to achieve the same sense of well-being, satiety, relaxation, and pain tolerance, all acting on fewer receptors for them.[109]

Preceding David Kessler, the gurus of the antisugar movement include Nancy Appleton, Kathleen DesMaisons, Joan Ifland, Anne Katherine, Kay Sheppard, and H. Leighton Steward. They devote the balance of their books to specific eating plans and some of them sneak in a twelve-step approach, with an agenda that is puritanical in comparison to other diets that allow points for a single-serving package of Oreos or a Skinny Cow ice cream sandwich. So puritanical is their

---

107   Angela Pirisi, "A Real Sugar High?," *Psychology Today* (January/February 2003).

108   Alcoholics Anonymous: Big Book, 4th ed. (Alcoholics Anonymous World Services, Inc., 2002), 133–34.

109   Kathleen DesMaisons, PhD, *Potatoes Not Prozac: Solutions for Sugar Sensitivity* (New York: Simon & Schuster, 1998).

approach, in fact, that they ban all of our beloved substitutes: aspartame (found in Equal and NutraSweet: good-bye Diet Coke), saccharin (Sweet'n Low), and cyclamate (Sugar Twin, which is scary stuff without the misgivings of Sheppard and Katherine, given that it carries the warning "Take only on the advice of a physician"). Sheppard's list of forbidden sweeteners is even more exhaustive, adding dextrose, maltodextrose, polydextrose, whey, syrups, malt, rice sweeteners, natural flavors (the Sheppard follower now proceeds to throw out her Celestial Seasonings Tuscan Orange Spice and Almond Sunset teas, among others), manitol, sorbitol, caramel color, artificial sweetener in packets. Packets probably includes sucralose, so now my favorite jam made with Splenda is off her grocery list, along with sugar-free Swiss Miss and Jell-O pudding.

Research backs up the omission of artificial sweeteners from these food plans. Rats at Purdue University that were fed yogurt sweetened with saccharin ate more than rats that ate natural glucose, although the saccharin-eaters' temperatures didn't rise as much, showing less active metabolisms.[110] Artificial sweeteners, while containing few calories, increase hunger and stimulate insulin, messing with the body in the same way as cane sugar.

Is this why the Angry Fat Girls have relapsed so often? Or did the other items on Kay Sheppard's prohibited food list lead us astray? I don't use a lot of the following, but I don't ban them, either: butter, sour cream, cream, cream cheese, dairy products over 2 percent fat, hard cheese, ricotta cheese, nuts, seeds, dried fruit, bananas, grapes, cherries, fruit juice, mangoes, popcorn, rice cakes, gum, chocolate, and caffeine.[111]

---

110 Ian Sample, "Sweetener May Increase Obesity Risk," *The Guardian* (UK), February 11, 2008.

111 Kay Sheppard, "The Food Plan," October 5, 2008, http://www.kaysheppard.com/foodplan.htm (accessed).

Katie would have gone to hell before breaking her McDonald's Diet Coke habit or Starbucks Venti with skim milk, which she considered sufficient for her breakfast dairy.

One of my sponsors had found recovery by staying at Kay's Place, Sheppard's in-home rehab. Monica has since relapsed and gone on to another twelve-step-based food plan, but when we talked about her eighteen months of living with *The Body Knows*,[112] she recalled wistfully her "beautiful, beautiful weight loss." Monica compared Sheppard's plan to the Bible: people take a piece of it and turn it into something so literal that you are straitjacketed into resenting everything else. "I used Crest when I was staying in Kay's home." She laughed. "It doesn't say anywhere that you have to use sugar-free toothpaste."

So why did Monica relapse? She'd been clean of sugar, flour, artificial sweeteners, and full-fat anything for more than 540 days straight. She'd lost sixty pounds. She was, more often than not, positively beaming with her new way of life.

One afternoon, at lunch with a close friend who knew about her food plan, Monica's cell phone rang. It was her oldest friend calling to tell her she had ovarian cancer that had metastasized in her liver and kidneys. Monica spoke supportively of treatments and booked a flight to Florida the next week. She told her lunch date about the crisis, picked up her plate, and went to the buffet. It took a long time to fill her plate because first she walked around the tables grabbing things—rolls, chicken wings, brownies, cubes of cheese, onion rings, fried wontons—as quickly and furtively as possible. Then she piled her plate high and gave her friend a look that said *don't go there* and dug in. A couple of days later, Monica walked into her very strict eating disorders group therapy session swigging from that equivalent

---

112 Kay Sheppard, *Food Addiction: The Body Knows* (Deerfield, FL: Health Communications, Inc., 1993).

of Pandora's Box, a twenty-ounce bottle of Diet Coke. She shrugged at her therapist and fellow analysands and broke down in sobs that were about her friend and whether she'd get kicked out of group but not about the brownies or the Cap'n Crunch cereal she'd eaten that morning.

She never got a sustained abstinence back, she regained her weight, and she lost not all of her belief in Kay Sheppard's food plan, but the essential spark that makes it work on a mental and physical level.

Monica may have already shot the moon running her own business that keeps her traveling, being a surrogate mother to her siblings, dealing with her own deep-seated grief at losing her mother at the age of twelve, and the death of her husband after less than a year of marriage. She may have laid all of her hormonal/neurotransmitter cards out on the table and been trumped with the news of the impending loss of her dearest friend and the extraordinary effort she would be exerting in escorting her caringly, lovingly, and with dignity from this world.

Had the promises of no cravings and an elevated mood failed in the face of sorrow and stress? And why, if that Baby Ruth candy bar has elevated my feel-good, feel-calm, feel-full serotonin levels, do I want three more?

None of the studies in addiction that I read addresses the possibility that people turn to and become dependent on sugar and refined carbohydrates because they don't manufacture or utilize enough of those feel-good chemicals *in the first place*. This is different from trying to feel "more better." It's an attempt to not feel the gray monotony of a chronic depression that has dogged some of us for as long as we can remember. Our brains were broken early. We live in a state of hopelessness, being pissed off, inadequacy, anxiety. We eat to forget, to get that serotonin-endorphin-dopamine chain gang pushing down the awareness of the bare existence we feel we live in.

"Perhaps you have fewer serotonin neurons than most people. Perhaps this condition was inherited . . . Perhaps the factory [at the neuron of tryptophan] isn't working well or maybe tryptophan isn't getting to the factory in sufficient quantities," author Anne Katherine hypothesizes from the findings of Benjamin Caballero published in the *International Journal of Obesity*.[113] Or, if I can offer a sugar addict's observation, increasing my sense of calm and well-being is more seductive than satiation or even engorgement. I eat more in order to feel less.

Once upon a time, I lost 188 pounds, got a new job at double my previous salary, sold a book for a respectable advance, received more than respectable reviews for it, had a couple of actual, well-meaning boyfriends, and overcame my fear of sweating in the public space of a gym. I couldn't stop crying. My psychiatrist put me on Zoloft and Wellbutrin. I weighed 150 pounds and I wasn't eating sugar. It had been four years, in fact, since I had eaten any but naturally occurring sugars and my limited amounts of saccharin. My psychiatrist has increased the dosages as we've gone along, adding Klonopin when my social anxiety became clearer to both of us.

What do you do when you've ceased self-medicating a depression that you were born with, gone on to change some huge negatives in your life, then moved on to prescribed medication because you're *STILL DEPRESSED*? I confess I don't know what Joan Ifland means when she swears, "We may still experience depression after replacing reactive foods, but it will be related to a real event, and not a chemical state."[114] Monica—and Katie and I, who are the Angry Fat Girls who have forsworn sugar and flour for long periods of time—ultimately reacted to real depression-spiking events the same way we did before we had twelve-step support and tools, therapists, antidepressants, and really cool clothes. The antisugar/anti–artificial sweetener pundits do not address what happens when the sugar addict gets clean, gets those

---

113 Katherine, 37.

114 Ifland, 7.

transmitters firing on their own or with psycho-pharmaceutical help, and still has patches of wanting to cry all day or crises that she can only deal with by reaching for the M&M's.

Late in January, in lieu of writing a real post on my personal blog, I copied and pasted the daily tenth step[115] inventory I did for my sponsor each night.

Lindsay, interested in the steps from the time she started reading about codependency, and so often the unwitting muse of this book, suggested that we all do the inventory on a closed blog. Wendy and Mimi agreed. We four had created the small phenomenon of Angry Fat Girlz and sharing how much we ate was sort of like being in a gym dressing room together—we already knew what jiggled when we were on the treadmill and what we looked like in bathing suits, so why be coy when changing our clothes? We deleted some questions that specifically pertained to my twelve-step program and added others that addressed problems we needed to work on.[116]

I asked to include Katie in the exercise. It would be good for her, I thought, to have more community and to look at what she accomplished each day rather than at the lifelong spectrum of what she regarded as her failures. She accepted our invitation but checked in only once to compliment us on our thoroughness and to apologize that she wasn't up to the task. I think she was frightened by giving away too much of

---

115 "Continued to take personal inventory and when we were wrong, promptly admitted it."

116 What did I eat today? What exercise did I have today? What did I do today that I like and respect myself for? (or How did I behave better than I felt?) What project was my priority for today and how much progress did I make on it? What do I plan to do next? What did I do for someone else today? What did I do for myself today? What happened today that I enjoyed and appreciated that had nothing to do with me? What boundaries did I set for myself? What boundaries did I honor? Where did I have problems today? (or Where did I feel bad or negative today?) What am I proudest of today? On a scale of one to ten, how much close interaction did I have with people today? What made me feel feminine today? What made me feel loved and appreciated today? What will I eat tomorrow?

herself and of the notes of encouragement, solace, and occasional bossi-
ness we posted on each other's entries. I think as well that her diffidence
about the inventory was the same diffidence she had about Lindsay,
Mimi, and Wendy. She could only trust one person at a time.

We shared days when our food was spot-on and days when we
train wrecked. On train-wreck days, we began to see, our lives had
not stopped and we had not stopped contributing to our individual
communities. My dogs still got exercised, and Wendy organized the
luncheon her boss was giving for the incoming dean of arts and sciences. Any one of us might have eaten Pop-Tarts, but there was clean
laundry and a really good book we finished reading and offered to
send off to a friend with similar interests. One of the riskiest issues
in losing weight was partially absolved in those sixteen questions. We
were more than what we ate. We were also hardworking, respected,
loved, observant, kind, intelligent, communal, and in process. And we
had friends who sympathized and gave gentle advice. I would wish
the feeling of the inventory's ongoing dialogue for anyone trying to
lose weight or see themselves beyond their weight.

Sometimes we fooled ourselves a little bit. Mimi was summoned
to Johns Hopkins on January nineteenth and twentieth for a series
of grueling interviews that included the director of Welch Library
and the director of emergency medicine, one of her areas of expertise.
She knew she'd done well and in answering "What did I do for *myself*
today?" she wrote that she "ordered French toast for breakfast instead
of a healthy one. I just wanted it—but I left some on the plate when I
was full." Being frank about our food was to recognize what was right
or wrong with it.

Our foibles revealed themselves day after day. I rarely dressed in
anything but sweatpants and hairy, holey sweaters, and often didn't
bathe for two or three days. Wendy could always find something to say
about feeling feminine, and if it wasn't about how much her clothes
cost it was, "my size 16 silk skirt and my size 18 jacket." Mimi revealed

the girliness that underlay her status as a wise woman: rabbits were bunnies, cats were kitties, her clinginess to anything pink. For Mimi and me, the peek into married life was fascinating if bewildering when Lindsay said she felt loved when Jalen told "me how good I looked in my workout clothes. Apparently sweaty is somehow sexy to him."

We illustrated our entries with images from the web or photos we'd taken. It had a scrapbook quality of four women who had decided to emerge from the shelter of their weight-loss programs, weight, dress sizes, or jobs. Writing our food down made what we were doing (or not doing) real to each other and to ourselves, and it made us take our daily lives beyond our food more seriously and self-consciously. Knowing we'd sit down to tell the stories of our days made us live more in the moment. Picking up a piece of trash or listening to a friend's boyfriend problems became more satisfying because we knew we'd write it up under "What did I do for someone else today?" We grasped at the shape of icicles or laughing babies to answer what we enjoyed that day. We also had the chance to see that we were more than the food we ate. Day by day, we had improved our worlds in small ways; we were supported by each other despite the Fritos; we could take pride in doing the laundry or calling our parents.

In anticipating the questions, we were forced to look around and be ready for the moment. It was an exercise in authenticity, and Lindsay was the most faithful writer.

Getting abstinent when I got back from Christmas in Arizona was a relief after being so out of control, but soon enough I found myself wanting a little night smackeral after the day's frustrations of dogs, the cold, and this book.

My book was, to borrow an expression from Wendy, stuck like white trash on Velveeta. I had three dozen interviews and a few pithy quotes, and I'd written two chapters about my relapse, but now I was reduced to writing figure eights, good technical feats but hardly the crowd-pleasing triple-lutz that wins medals.

I raged about this to Lindsay in our morning phone calls. "I'm a funny writer," I said. "I'm a personal writer. I have no credentials to give advice about this or that."

She agreed. Those were the things that had drawn her to me through *Passing for Thin*.

"I've got all this crap about how regaining weight is the perfect Aristotelian tragedy. I'm gonna scrap it. That's the only thing I know I'm going to do writingwise. What about you?"

"I need to transcribe an interview with a guy who used to be the editor of the *Texas Observer*. He had great stuff on Ann Richards. I'm working at IT today, so I can only do a little after work, but I can start."

One of the things I admired about Lindsay and Wendy was that they didn't binge work or binge procrastinate. They knew how to put twenty minutes on the elliptical trainer or in getting the first five minutes of an interview onto paper and then move on. I seemed to need wide blocks of time to do anything, and I approached work—writing or walking dogs—with such a pounding heart and nervous stomach that I usually took half a Klonopin in order not to jump out of my skin. I wouldn't need chemical calm that Thursday. Deleting how spectacle and diction help make the woman who regains weight a tragic heroine wasn't a challenge. It was merely pathetic.

Another tombstone-skied day. Lindsay called, huffing against the cold as she walked to campus. "So how cool is it that Mimi got the job?"

"I'm *so* excited for her," I said. Mimi had emailed everyone she'd ever known the day before with the news that she'd been hired with a hefty raise by Welch Medical Library. "We should send flowers."

"Good idea. Can you order them and let me know how much to send you?"

"Yeah. I'll ask Wendy if she's in . . . or I'll just add her name. Lindsay and Mimi have never gotten to know each other, have they?"

"I think Katie's anger scares her," Lindsay said. "Katie probably thinks Mimi's a wuss."

"More like a mystery," I answered. "'What's behind that smile?'"

"So what kind of flowers should we send?"

"Ummm . . . wild guess here, but what about . . . *pink*?"

Lindsay huffed a laugh and changed the subject. "She and Wendy are hooked on *Clean House*. I think they're in a competition now. Wendy didn't realize this was gonna mean furniture."

"You know they're only a couple of hours away from each other, don't you?" I asked. "Wendy will be able to hoard *New Yorker*s and take them up to Mimi."

"And Mimi can load her down with newt-foot candles and romance novels," she said, and then gave a long sigh. "I *have* to get this dissertation done. Mimi got the job of her dreams. It's a sign. I'll get the next job if I finish my dis."

"I just want to tell stories," I said with a heavier sigh.

"But whose?"

"Ours."

I blinked with surprise. Of course I'd intended to use Mimi and Lindsay, Katie and Wendy among the interviews I'd done, but I hadn't thought of using them almost exclusively.

"Ours?"

"The AFGs'. I can't stand the thought of writing one of those thesis-case-in-point books. You know: 'Some people can't stop eating. Sally was one of those people. She was born blah-blah-blah . . .' I think I'll die of boredom if I have to write like that. I want to write a novel."

"But, Frances, you didn't sell a novel."

"Not a fiction novel. A nonfiction novel." How many query letters had I tossed immediately upon seeing that stupid phrase when I was an agent? Thousands, I guessed. "Like *In Cold Blood*, only not. About us, the people I know."

"Can you change a few things?" she asked cautiously. "I mean, we have jobs and parents and . . . husbands."

"Yeah," I said, thinking fast. "I can do that. But we need to meet. We've computed and cell phone conferenced and Christmas carded ourselves to smithereens. I need to put faces on words."

"Hmm. A convention. Interesting."

Could I pull it off? Could I stay abstinent until they came and stay abstinent while they were here? I'd lived on an iceberg with my dogs and writing and fat: Could I step off it in order to spend sustained time with people? That need to be present was why I ate when I went to see my parents, the prison of boredom that comes from their infirmities and their airless, eventless retirement community, my fear of losing them, my fear that they will suck me dry.

And yet, it was thrilling. I'd found the key to this book through the stories we had assembled in every way but being together. I felt like I finally had fire in my belly, and, as Katie and Mimi and then Wendy said yes, I felt like I finally had sisters.

As if she had read my mind, late in January, two weeks into her glowing new-old abstinence, Katie wrote a blog about what weighing, as she put it, "in excess of four hundred bills" had cost her:

Being able to do stand-up comedy
Being able to join an improv group
Writing comedy
Following my dream of working as a comedian
The ability to go to any show I want
The ability to go to any activity
The ability to care for myself in a natural way
The ability to go for a walk
The ability to form a lasting partnership with another human
     being
The ability to have a job
The ability to add to society

The ability to go on a trip
The ability to find clothes that fit
The ability to find shoes that fit
The desire to dress becomingly
Respect for myself

"I notice that a lot of these missing areas of my life involve 'ability,'" she observed. "That is what this disease has taken from me: ability."

As I started my own day, wearing fetid down ski pants and a sweater that was more dog hair than wool, I was grateful that I could mostly still *go*. I had miles of walking in a whiplash of windchill that day; I could take a shower or get on a plane without going first class. But I had nothing like Katie's dreams of the work and fun she so specifically wanted. What was that about? I wondered. I'd always been a dreamer.

I'd had dreams once—to be thin, to write and publish a book, to fall mutually and sanely in love—but I achieved the first two and came to understand the last was out of my control and required enormous effort and strength. Having had the same dreams for the better part of forty-three years, I had never really bulked up the skill of dreaming.

We tell ourselves we must lose weight in order to be there for our kids to grow up, to look good, to find a mate, to get our mothers' approval, to get a better job. These may be the motivations for wanting to lose weight but I've come to think that motivation should be removed from the weight-loss vocabulary. Having a reason is too finite for the task of losing many pounds and maintaining that success. Our kids turn into snotty preteens, and we use food to control our tempers and, a little, to have revenge. We get the job and then get complacent. You'd think we'd get it that losing weight has to be about something bigger than ourselves, and yet I hear it all the time: *I want to be thin for my daughter's wedding* or *my twentieth reunion is coming up.* The dieter either gives up because she realizes she won't fit the fantasy evening gown in time or she gets down to her cheerleader uniform size but eats the entire breakfast buffet.

Shame, by contrast, is a more powerful motivation. Every dieter should keep her shame green. After manifold dropouts from Weight Watchers, what Betsy saw when she looked in the mirror propelled her to a surgeon. I disgust myself when I hide my shame by taking my binge boxes to a building where I'm dog-sitting and putting them in their recycling bin. But shame is a running away from rather than a running to, and the latter is the sweetness of what we think about before falling asleep at night.

Dreams were one of the missing weapons in Lindsay's, Mimi's, Wendy's, and my year of trying to lose weight. Lindsay wanted to finish her dissertation and get a teaching job, and Mimi was pleased and proud of her new position at John Hopkins, but these were desires, like thirst. They were finite and accomplishable within a wide weight range. Wendy wrote on her original questionnaire that her dream was to be a writer, but I think her capacity for independent balls-to-the-wind action was robbed by a silent, fuzzy childhood controlled by a controlling and violent father and a pessimistic, belittling mother. Imprisonment is her default setting.

Mimi's original questionnaire says that her dream is to be a web designer, but this is as finite and removed from weight as her new job. Had her ability to dream big been squelched by parents who supported her through an excellent education that came with the understanding that her degrees had to lead to supporting herself? A husband, art, vagabondism were implicitly negated in that contract.

My own dream mechanisms were broken. Three years earlier, when I put on my favorite size 6 suit and handed in the final draft of *Passing for Thin*, I didn't know that I didn't know how to replace the Weird Sisters that had evaded me for so long and left me spinning when their prophecies came true. Now the question was how could I kick my imagination into giving me the infinite horizon I needed in order to re-lose eighty pounds and build a life I loved? I had no answers except to mumble, *If only I wasn't so depressed, I could figure it out. If only I wasn't so cold. If only I wasn't so fat.*

Of all of us, Katie was the only one who lived in the clouds. Perhaps that's the one great legacy her gambler father left her. I never brushed her off as too fantastical. Indeed, I urged her to find classes to study comedy. Her dreams could save her if she found the path to a healthy, mobile weight.

And I needed to sound my heart plumb for the impossibilities from which I could next reinvent myself.

Maybe by writing a nonfiction novel.

TWELVE

March

The Angry Fat Girls

As the brutality of the winter of 2006 continued into March, as our plans to meet morphed and codified, facts and truths began to merge.

Some of the facts were uncomfortable. It was a sign of Wendy's relative mental health and certainly her unending generosity that, early in the Amazon blog days, she had reached out to Katie with support and offers of clothes she'd shrunk out of. Katie didn't reciprocate beyond polite thanks. Katie prefers to discover friends rather than be found, a quirk of many parts. She doesn't believe she's worth being picked out of a crowd, for one. And by being the chooser, she unconsciously looks for people as much and as unhealthily in need of an obsessive friendship as she is. Remember: Katie chose me by volunteering to be interviewed. Our friendship was a healthy one because I knew the facts and the truth about her and her ailments.

The AFGs always asked about Katie, in phone calls and email, and Katie asked about them. They were mutually curious and already had fixed ideas about each other with very little contact except through each other's personal blogs. Mimi found Katie's anger frightening, and Katie laughed cruelly at Mimi's Wiccan convictions. Wendy was a little hurt by Katie's rebuff, and Katie thought Wendy was a silly little girl. Lindsay gave the least thought to Katie, and vice versa. They were worlds apart in where they were in their own lives.

But Katie was important to me and the story I had gone back and begun to reassemble. Instead of eating, we'd spend hours on the phone whittling away Saturday nights in chat, gossip, confessions, twelve-step talk, and stories. She was thrilled with her Christmas presents and cried when she realized the Anne Taintor dish cloth she got in the mail a day or two after moving into her new apartment was a housewarming token from me. "No one's ever done anything like that for me," she emailed.

To the AFGs' consternation, I invited Katie. She considered what it would be like to come and her requirements weren't easy.

"I would love to go see a show, but I'm afraid I might have trouble with the seats," Katie said. "It would take coordination to get me handicapped seating. I can't do a ton of walking with you all, which is why I'm skeptical if I should come." She had broken into the three hunskies—the three C-notes, Benjamins, yards—and was feeling physically better at 396. She could buy groceries, take them to the car, unload them, and put them away without having to stop and sit down. But New York is a city of stairs, sidewalks, and waiting in lines, and she'd have to negotiate luggage, Oakland International, and JFK first. Wistfully, Katie decided not to come. With equal wistfulness, I wondered if I could get out to San Francisco. She was ambivalent: I'd have to be abstinent, we couldn't do much, it would cost a lot of money. We tabled the conversation for another time, which never came.

One of the rhythms of the AFGs is the academic calendar and mid-March was spring break for everyone else. I was boarding out with Italian greyhounds for ten days, which meant the Bat Cave, which can sleep two, was free. I found a couch with friends and suddenly we had dates and free rooming.

I went blotto OCD. I needed washcloths to match my towels. The temperature dials of my stove could only be cleaned with Q-tips. My pillows needed dry cleaning. How was I going to pull off playing tour guide? Personalities emerged as real things to contend with instead of hang up on. Wendy emailed me on the QT to say she'd like some alone time or possibly to stay longer in order to go to the Met and to the Neue Galerie. There was a whiff of the invidious in addressing me privately, an implication that no one else would be highbrow enough to want to look at Klimts. She'd been to New York once and considered herself an old hand. Her suggestions for Lindsay, the neophyte, were bizarrely similar to those of Katie's boyfriend who wanted to have his picture taken with the cardboard cutout of George Costanza.

"She's so political," she reasoned. "Don't you think she'd get a kick out of the NBC Store?" I was silently amused. The NBC Store was one of the places she'd hit on her one one-day trip to New York.

Wendy got it half-right. Lindsay's politics could be fostered in the city. "I kind of want to see *The Daily Show*, but I'm not married to the idea," she emailed me as I fretted and scrubbed dishes with S.O.S. pads. I have place settings for at least eight people; however, all but one had turned yellow with disuse. "I'm coming to meet you guys. Whatever we do is fine."

Whatever we do is fine: I hate those words. It's a fat thing: I *need* people I'm traveling with or entertaining to have a good time so that they'll a) forget what I look like, b) forget the weakness and slothfulness that I am, and c) be in debt to me, a fat person's approximation of love. To make it all worse, I, a fat woman, was in charge of three fat women. The Fat Code would be in complete effect. No one would voice an opinion, a desire, a dislike, an objection. We'd look like a collection of bobble-head dolls, always deferring, always listening for the subtle code of disagreement: "If that's what you want to do . . ." "Whatever you say . . ." "I'm just along for the ride . . ."

If I were a generous person, I'd say that's why Wendy was so confidential about extra time for fine art—she couldn't stand the guilt of imposition on the rest of us.

My actual generosity teamed up with my love of eBay, and I went shopping for welcome presents.

A flying pig pin in pink sparkles for Mimi. She could wear it with anything, and it would be a part of her collection and the never-say-never hopes she had never articulated to me.

Celtic wolf head earrings for Lindsay, who explained her choice of totem as "No special reason . . . I think my personality is sort of dog-like—open and friendly but with a mean twist if I'm threatened. I'm also very protective of people I care about. And my Chinese astrology sign is the dog."

A polar bear wearing a cat bracelet for Wendy. She loved the roly-poly playfulness of polar bears and the antics of her cats, Miss Bucket ("That's *'Bouquet'* ") and Iago, that were often the sole answer to "What did I enjoy today that had nothing to do with me?"

An Indian elephant pendant for Katie, whom I wanted to include as much as I could. Her identification with elephants was as much about their loyalty and capacity for sadness as it was about their size.

These are their self-chosen totem animals. I decided to go Mimi one better in the realm of ceremonies and gods, and make some aspects of the meeting ritualistic. Our animal allies would protect us.

I didn't buy a new totem for myself, a grizzly bear or penguin something, any more than I would have bought a present for myself when shopping for someone's birthday. The colony of penguins living in the Bat Cave is reminiscent of my grade school nuns, although they failed to inspire me to mate, dress well, eat more fish, or take the occasional water slide. The grizzly is the state animal of Montana. I have a pair of grizzly paw earrings that I wear when I'm not in the mood to take any shit and intend that things are going to go my way. How gracious would that attitude be?

There were two things I announced we would do: go to the Met to figure out what it means to be Rubenesque and hold a burning ceremony, a twelve-step thing, in which we would write down the flaws and obsessions we are ready to let go of and then burn them. I asked my sponsor, Patty, to be our witness and the AFGs agreed she was probably the perfect and only outsider we could invite for such a weird moment.

Whatever else they wanted to do, I was ... um ... happy to go along for the ride.

I had placed highly in the Christmas weight gain lottery, but our plans invigorated my resolve and by early March I had a six-week run of abstinence going when I met Pam Peeke for dinner at a swank hotel on the East Side. Pam scares the shit out of me: she's a force of nature, a Valkyrie played by Annie Lennox. Without pausing for breath, she enumerated the people she'd met with in New York in the last twenty-four hours and then switched to firing off questions to me.

"So. What are you up to these days?"

"Oh ... writing. Walking dogs." I had exactly two notes to my scale.

"How's the dog thing?"

I smiled. "They're fabulous. They keep me laughing."

She narrowed her eyes speculatively. "How much do you think you'd weigh without the dogs?"

Now there was a poser I'd rather not have had to think about.

"Three hundred pounds," I said off the top of my head. "It's not so much the exercise as not being able to eat sugar during the day. I'm too dopey for four big hostile dogs if I eat sugar."

She nodded as though I'd confirmed a detail in a draft of a National Institute of Health article she was writing.

"How's the book going? How's it going to end?" She dug into her salmon.

"The women the book is about are coming to visit in a couple of weeks," I answered. "I won't know until they give me the ending."

She fixed me with her gimlet stare. Pam wouldn't need a scalpel to perform surgery. She could just *stare* a tumor out of a patient. "Bullshit."

"What do you mean? They're the story."

"*You're* the story." She took me in: the dinner I'd ordered (baked chicken), what I was wearing (black wool trousers and blazer), the size of me. "You're the brand, kiddo. You owe your readers a happy ending."

I was suddenly very glad I had not shared her crab quesadilla starter, and I was pretty sure I'd be stopping for ice cream when I walked Daisy later. Whatever my story was going to be that night, I wanted it to be a quick private escape.

It was a fine early spring Tuesday when I met Mimi's train at Penn Station. She was the first to arrive. Hero, one of the Labs that often hung out in the Bat Cave during the day, hovered shyly around the fuss but Daisy was ecstatic at her new auntie. She ran to the love seat and whapped her tail and scraped the air with her right paw, inviting Mimi to come and sit, then promptly collapsed on her and twisted over for a belly rub, her amber eyes confident.

"Oh, come let us adore me," I sang to the tune of "O Come All Ye Faithful." "I'm Dai-sy the Dog." Mimi laughed. Two hours later, when Lindsay turned up, she taught the song to her.

Well after the visit, Lindsay shared her impressions of the three of us, my apartment, Brooklyn Heights, the city, and my [ha ha] leadership. Certain things stood out as comfortable and right, and others as uncomfortable and confusing.

I thought you were pissed off when you met me at the front door. You wouldn't look me in the eye, and your face seemed frozen under these fierce eyebrows. I'd read and heard so much about about the Bat Cave, and I was curious to see it. It was as dark as you said it was, and as tiny. I couldn't look at the bookcases and pictures, but I felt like there was another crowd waiting beyond the people and excited dogs.

No one believes that I—tell-all memoirist, sweat-free on the set of the *Saturday Today Show*, lecturing two hundred vegans on the evils of sugar—am intensely shy. I looked unapproachable when I was actually worrying about what Lindsay would think of me and my apartment, whether she liked dogs in person or liked them as an idea. As she hugged Mimi hello and Daisy introduced herself, I had a chance to take her in as she took my tiny sanctuary in. I hadn't noticed that she needed orthodontia for her pigeon-toed front teeth, and she could have benefited from a good haircut. She was thin but not skinny, and not as pretty as I'd built her up to be.

At that, I relaxed a fraction and announced that I had to collect Boomer and walk Hero home. I invited them to come along—I'd take the dogs down to the Promenade and Lindsay would get her first sight of how unfathomable the glass citadel of Lower Manhattan is.

I'm sure Lindsay was relieved when we hit the sunny sidewalk on our way to Boomer's house, glad to be out of the tiny, crowded cubby that is my home.

Mimi admitted that she was tired after strolling the twenty-two blocks that brought us, Daisy, and Boomer back to my front door. I suggested they take some time to unpack and unwind while I took Boomer home and went off to feed Daisy and the Mighty Mites, the greyhounds Daisy and I were staying with. I lay on the couch and worried about where to take Mimi and Lindsay for dinner, what we should do that night. I had three days to introduce Lindsay to New York and Mimi's bad knees to factor in.

Times Square, I thought, despite how much I hate the crowds and how suddenly tired I felt. This meant two sets of stairs, plus an elevator and escalator on the Seventh Avenue subway. Mimi could do it, and Times Square was one of those things you had to see in order to understand how three New Yorks function at once: the neighborhoods, the capital of commerce, and touristy fun town.

How many of the thousands of people there that night found

irony in the triangulation of an M&M fanning his arms in a "ta-da: the show ends here," and Mr. Peanut tipping his hat at the mega-lighted pile of Twizzlers, Mounds and Heath Bars, Reese's cups and York Peppermint Patties on top of the Hershey's store? If we bought one of each snack shining against the night and shared it, we'd have eaten more than a thousand calories.

When Daisy and I came home from Chez Mighty Mites the next morning, I saw that Lindsay had twisted the light on the desk to read. The shade on my bedside lamp had disintegrated and all that was left was a spindly old stand and a bare sixty-watt bulb. "I wanted to read a little to unwind. The glare was awful," she explained.

I wondered if it was as awful as I felt for having overlooked another piece of my crappy house.

Mimi tucked her CPAP machine in its bag and looked around at the little boxes and photos, books and dolls, and the dogs' plush toys. "I could never live here. I need much more space than this."

Lindsay added, "Bat Cave Rule Number One: Don't put anything down. You'll never find it."

"Okay." I laughed. "Is there anything you *like* about my house?" They giggled. "It's *very* New York," Lindsay said. "It never really gets dark, even in the Cave, where it's dark in the daytime. And I was startled by the sound coming up from the floor. Then I realized it was the subway. I like the feeling of so much life, going on all around us. All I had to do was hope I didn't dream about nuns and M&M's all night." "Lindsay was threatening to turn on all the lights and count your nuns," Mimi said. "How many do you have, anyway? They're even in the kitchen."

"It would have taken all night," Lindsay said, "and I'd already set my mental alarm clock for 'early' so I could take a walk around the neighborhood at my own speed, then read my book over the biggest cup of coffee to be had and a fresh hot bagel at that little place on the main street."

Mimi smiled benignly. "And I slept in. We both got what we wanted." She reached and picked up a little blue enamel box, opened it and inspected its contents of paper clips. "I could never live here," Mimi said. "But you know, as crammed as the Bat Cave is in the day-time, it has a womblike quality at night."

"And now?" I asked.

"The next morning, the Bat Cave has no breakfast in it."

As I led them off to my favorite diner, I thought about them nest-ling into the pillows and quilts and I knew that just as Lindsay's eyes grew too heavy to keep open, Mimi would have said softly, as she had to me so many nights on the phone, "Good night, lovey. Sweet dreams." I wished I'd been there.

Lindsay busted into the Bat Cave in triumph.

"Two pairs of shoes!" she said excitedly. "That is a fabulous shop." She stopped short and looked at Wendy, playing Scrabble on my computer. "Wendy! Hi!"

"Hi! It's good to see you—"

The word *again* hung in the air like a balloon. Everyone laughed and the moment passed. This was going to be fine, I thought to myself. Each of us had thought the same thing—that we were already so familiar with each other that Lindsay's skipped "It's good to meet you" was completely natural. No one felt compelled to say this out loud.

"You've *got* to see these shoes!" Lindsay said.

Wendy towered over Lindsay and diminutive Mimi when she stood up for the unveiling. Rawboned and thick-haunched, she made me feel small, which is saying something. I'm five foot eight and that day, I weighed 220 pounds. Wendy's need to watch our lips was unnerving, and I wondered how much she hadn't heard already.

"Ooooh . . ." she cooed. "You got them around here?"

"Did you pay cash and get the discount?" I asked.

"No, and I pretty much shot my wad for the trip, but look!"

"They're gore-jus," Wendy said. Her speech was slightly thick, with a tinny upper register, and her drawl was as prodigious in person as it was on the phone. "Can we go there? Now?"

"Of course!" Lindsay laughed happily. "Shoe shopping is better than therapy! And the owner asked me how long I've lived in the Heights! Isn't that cool? You're gonna love this neighborhood, Wendy. It's so homey."

"I already do," Wendy said. "It's like I fell into an Edith Wharton novel."

I scratched Daisy's ears as they headed out to look at shoes on Montague Street. They were happy. I had one last dog walk and then I'd take Wendy over to my friends' house. If all went well, I'd be in bed by nine o'clock.

The next morning, Mimi and Lindsay told Wendy and me about their excursion to the Empire State Building.

"I hope you're not pissed off that we went without you," Lindsay said.

"It was a last-minute decision," Mimi added, "and it was eight thirty. We know Frances goes to bed at sunset, and I didn't want to disturb Wendy's hosts by her coming in late."

"That's okay," Wendy said in the three-note singsong that suggested she was forgiving rather than understanding them. Then again, Wendy had said all along that she was keen on museums rather than tourist sights.

I was relieved. They'd done a big New York Thing and I hadn't had to endure the wait.

"How long was the line?" I asked.

"Long. My back hurt," Mimi admitted. "My knees hurt. But it was fun." She slapped the menu down. "I want French toast. What are you guys having?"

"Whatever you do," I said, "you have to have the potato pancakes. Teresa's is famous for them."

"Then I'll have a Cheddar cheese omelet," Lindsay decided. "With a cinnamon raisin bagel."

"And I'll have the Swiss cheese omelet," I said.

Wendy had waited us out and continued to study the menu. "Maybe Ah'll just have the fruit since we're getting potato pancakes."

Lindsay groaned and looked at Mimi to do the dirty work.

"We're not counting points, Wen. Order what you want."

"D'y'all think it's too early for chicken livers and french fries?"

Mimi made a face of distaste but laughed. "I was worried about whether everyone was going to count my points, too."

"I've been too hungry to even really look at what anyone else is eating." Lindsay laughed.

"Did you know there are ten million bricks in the Empire State Building?" Mimi said as she reached into her bag for her camera. She turned it on and handed it to Wendy to scroll through the pictures. There she was, my twinkling city. Mimi had zoomed in on the Verrazano Bridge, the lovely double-strand of jade; on the Brooklyn Bridge, a rope of diamonds; on the Manhattan Bridge, sapphires and pearls. The Chrysler Building poked its churchy spire out of the other million lights. The city was like the most elegant cocktail dress, black, gold, pale green.

Last of all was a picture of Lindsay, her hair blowing in the wind, her black T-shirt showing a sliver of belly, her shirt and blazer meeting in a rectangle of cleavage. She is smiling and has the languid, sleepy sexiness of Jane Russell.

She looked as proud and pleased in that photo as the skyscraper itself.

Thursday boded a change of weather and it had begun to rain when we left my favorite Szechuan dive at the end of Canal Street. We had to trudge down to Grand Street before I could hail a cab. I opened the front passenger door and suggested Mimi would be more comfortable there and Wendy, Lindsay, and I smashed ourselves together in the backseat. It was every fat woman's nightmare—and every not-so-fat woman's as well, it turned out. "The thing I remember most," Lindsay told me months later, "was how big you all were. You were all hunched up and only spoke to give directions."

"Because if we pinched ourselves together and didn't breathe, we might seem smaller," I told her.

Mimi's face pinched a little more when we got out and saw the broad, long sweep of steps up to the Metropolitan Museum. When she came to New York for my birthday, we'd taken cabs to flat places. It had not prepared her, or her two replaced knees, for what we were doing on this trip.

I cringed at what I was making her do but tried to remind myself that you'd have to be dead not to love *something* in the Met, even if she or the others found themselves bored witless by the Rubenses.

It was a choice, when we left the lurid seventeenth-century Spanish painters behind us, between the *The Feast of Acheloüs* and *Venus and Adonis*. *The Feast of Acheloüs* is a cacophonous, sensual, bucolic version of *The Last Supper*, with three or four female nudes framing the central event. *Venus and Adonis* is three figures, of which the naked Venus is the most prominent. We chose Venus because she was the only woman in the painting and we could study her without the distraction of comparisons. It was also a more familiar story. The tragedy that was about to unfold was in the tensed muscles and gloomy forest behind Adonis, Venus, and Cupid.

We sat down on two of the benches and basked in it.

Our eyes were drawn first to Venus clutching Adonis's arm to keep him from going to the hunt. They traveled up to her face next, taking in her cherry mouth and flow of curls, then down to the chubby Cupid clutching Adonis's leg. Only then did we zero in on Adonis's perfectly captured sort of galumphy youth and on Venus's strong legs and dimpled knees.

Her knees that are the real deal, the signature of the twenty-first century's definition of a "weight problem" and unacceptability.

"What size do you think she is?" I asked.

"An eighteen?" Mimi hazarded.

"I'm a size eighteen and she looks smaller than me," I said doubtfully.

"I looked like her when I was a sixteen," Lindsay said with some harshness. "I hated it."

"But look at her, she's beautiful," I protested. Venus is no wimp in Rubens's painting, but she is vulnerable. Her face is pleading but flawlessly pale with just the right blush of carnal vigor in her cheeks. In fact, she looked a lot like Mimi if Mimi had long curly hair. "Did you even *look* at your body then?" I went on.

"Yes. I would stand in front of the mirror and pick out every little flaw."

Lindsay was adamant. She had shown herself to be the most balanced, the most emotionally and physically healthy, of us, not because she was thinner than us, but because she had built the certainty of grappling with difficulties into her life. That commitment to struggle was part of what made Lindsay a whole person. A tough marriage, yes, but she supported Jalen's exercise addiction recovery wholeheartedly and took a searching look at her part in supporting his addiction. She loved her field of study and dissertation topic, was close to her family, went to parties thrown by friends or colleagues, had lunch every week with a close girlfriend, owned a home and planted flowers, attended her Spiritualist Church each week, came alive ten minutes into a run. I wasn't jealous of her, but I was envious of how many quilt blocks her life was made up of and how well stitched together they were.

"And yet no one would say, 'Venus could stand to lose a few,'" Mimi said.

"Was it social pressure that made you hate your body then?" I pushed Lindsay.

"No. I just did. I hated the bits and pieces, the bulges. I thought I was ugly."

"Venus has lumpy thighs." It was hard to tell whether Wendy was adding this to the discussion of Lindsay's Rubenesque past or whether she couldn't hear us and made an observation on her own.

"That's all right for Venus," Lindsay said. "But I wanted a straight up and down body."

"Like a size ten?" I asked.

"Yes. Like everybody else."

"So it *was* societal expectations," I trumped her.

"Yes and no. I just wasn't comfortable at a size sixteen."

There was silence as we studied the painting further. Sadly, Wendy said, "She has ankles."

"I have ankles." I pull up the legs of my jeans.

Wendy and Mimi did the same. They had fence posts for ankles.

"But she has a waist," I hastened to add. "Wendy has a waist."

"She looks a lot older than Adonis," Wendy said.

"Yeah, well, she's a *goddess*," Mimi protested. "She *was* older. Lots and lots older."

"But the discrepancy in ages is really apparent," Wendy said. "And Cupid is pretty chubby, too. It looks like Adonis really wants to get away from them."

"Codependency or death?" I asked. "That was his choice."

"When I was a sixteen, I didn't have perky breasts or toned arms. She really fills her body out," Lindsay said.

"She's a goddess. Rubens might make her big, but he's not going to give her droopy tits," I answered.

"True. But the rest of her seems true to life. Big ass and thighs, smaller waist, broad shoulders, muscular arms."

"Some people think Rubens's women arc like that because he used male models for his paintings," Mimi told us. "She doesn't look like she's based on a male body, though. She's got muscles in the right places and her fat is fat, not muscle."

Wendy stood up and looked toward the jolly Hals and Watteaus that waited us. "Have you noticed that none of his nude women have nipples?"

We laughed and stood up. I needed to say hello to Caravaggio's musicians, as beautiful as Adonis without his callowness, their corruption forced on them before they knew they were innocent rather than by the seduction of an almost-man who had only that skill left to learn.

By the time I got back from feeding the greyhounds, a hard wind had kicked up and the temperature was falling. Patty had arrived and Wendy, Mimi, and Lindsay had gone on strike against letting me pay for more meals. Tired and weather-weary, we agreed without words not to go back into the city for dinner after our burning ceremony.

Patty is the size and vividness of a hummingbird, likely to show up in emerald and rose, with a slash of amethyst for good measure. She is, always, a student, a little kerfuffled by the practicalities of life but absorbing the mysteries without trying to slot them into categories. At my best, I inspired her, and at my worst, I worried her a lot.

"So why are you in an eating disorders program?" Lindsay was saying as I came in. "You're—*skinny*." The word wasn't necessarily a compliment.

"There are many ways to abuse yourself with food," Patty said, and told them a little of her history.

"Hardcore, huh?" I asked as I fished around for pens and paper. Mimi would understand the ceremony as a cleansing, Lindsay as a freeing of the spirit. I agreed with the validity in their interpretations and, as a Catholic who knows how pagan her church essentially is, saw it as an oblation, sacrament, and intention all rolled into one nutty bit of theology.

I had wanted to burn our faults over the East River, letting the fire and ashes flow into the water and its ocean-bound currents, going for as many of the four elements as my patch of Brooklyn allowed, but the night was turning ugly. I couldn't see putting Mimi through the twenty-block trip with a steep hill that would take us to Fulton Landing.

"The Promenade," I said. "Nobody's going to be there and there's plenty of air and water now."

Lindsay plucked the paper lei hanging from my desk lamp and put it on Daisy's head. "Daisy will be our Good Fairy," she said. "The one with no evil in her, dressed in the earth." We laughed at the lop-sided crown she wore with dignified aplomb.

We hadn't anticipated how hard it would be to get increasingly dampening paper to catch fire in the rain and wind. My thumb was singed and abraded from trying to keep my lighter lit. "We should give up," I said after five minutes of this. "We can tear them up into little bits and throw them in the trash." As we headed down the Pierrepont exit from the Promenade, my hair stopped whipping my eyes. I tried my lighter again. The slight shelter of bushes and trees by the play-ground was enough of a windbreak to keep it lit. One by one, we fed our desires into the flame, sometimes with an "Oh, shit!" when the wind caught the ragged burn and tore it into sudden flame.

And then it was over. I'd burned my plea to the elements to relieve me of my unquenchable desire for sugar, so crazed by managing four guests and my dog, the inclement night, the lighter, the need to feed the greyhounds, that what looked like my solemnity was distraction. I was anywhere and everywhere but in my own heart as my piece of paper caught fire and threatened to travel up my sleeve.

"Should we pray?" Patty asked.

There was a confounded silence until Lindsay said, "How about the Spiritualist Prayer of Healing?"

Patty's face lit up in interest. "What is it?" she asked eagerly.

Lindsay cleared her throat. "Repeat after me: 'I ask the Great Unseen Healing Force to remove all obstructions from my mind and body and to restore me to perfect health. I ask this in all sincerity and honesty, and I will do my part. I ask this Great Unseen Healing Force to help both present and absent ones who are in need of help and to restore them to perfect health. I put my trust in the power and love of God.'"

Only the wind and the rain spoke when we finished. I thought of Katie, probably getting around to weighing and measuring her lunch as we stood on the Promenade, of the readers of our blogs, of Lindsay's uncle gimping around on his new prosthesis, of all the people I'd seen come and go or come and stay in the Rooms. I knew each of us was thinking along the same lines. I wanted to cry but the Zoloft/Wellbutrin barrier made it hard, and I had so much to do before bed.

We woke, in our separate domiciles, to snow. As the day warmed slightly, the snow turned to rain. The airports were a mess. Lindsay was frantic about her flight early the next morning, and her airline wasn't reassuring her when she called every half hour. She was aching for Jalen and wanted a good night's sleep and an anonymous departure. She also wanted a good shower. My bathtub had decided that draining was too much work for its antique pipes. I'd caught Lindsay and Mimi with a bottle of Liquid-Plumr, imploring the water to move. They were chagrined that I walked in on them, but I was horrified at one of my shames being exposed.

Late that afternoon I put Lindsay in a town car bound for a Wall Street hotel she'd found online at a bargain price. It pulled away from the curb and kicked a nice spray of slush onto my pants. It was getting colder. The rain was turning to sleet. By the time I returned from feeding the greyhounds, we were in the middle of an ice storm.

"Do you think Lindsay's going to make it out tomorrow?" I asked Mimi as I hung up my coat.

"Lindsay will find a way. She'll get out and kick the plane into the air if she needs to."

We laughed. Because she was the thinnest and youngest of us, we had naturally deferred to Lindsay, and as an oldest child and wife of a passive, somewhat lost man, she accepted her leadership without noticing.

Mimi's cell phone rang. She said hello, followed by a very long silence as she listened intently. "Oh, my God," she said. "You've gotta talk to Frances."

Wendy had gone down to the Promenade to take pictures of the ice on all the black wrought iron. She slipped and knew as she fell that something had gone terribly wrong with her right knee. People rushed over to help her but she shushed them away, pulled out her cell phone, and dialed 911. A man ran back to his car and brought a blanket for her. Two women stood by and waited until the ambulance came, trying to reassure her that everything would be okay. Wendy looked dolefully at her swelling pant leg and tried to thank them for their time and concern.

"Hey," she said gaily, "at least I'll be able to say I've seen the inside of a New York City ER. There're some real characters here."

It was Saturday night, the eve of St. Patrick's Day. I shuddered to think what kind of characters were drifting in.

"Have you seen a doctor?"

"Yeah." She sighed. "He cut my jeans up the side. My favorite Gap size twenty jeans. I'm more pissed off about that than I am at falling."

"What did he say?"

"He took an X-ray. He doesn't think anything's broken, but I'm waiting for him to come back. He says I can't walk on it."

There was no way I was skating to Long Island Hospital on nine blocks of black ice. I called the car service through which I'd dispatched Lindsay to Manhattan and was told that because of the road conditions, it would be a thirty-dollar trip and an additional five dollars for every ten minutes they had to wait for me to retrieve Wendy. Lindsay had crossed the Brooklyn Bridge for less than fifteen dollars. I was dismayed at the price until we started our skittering progress toward Amity Street.

After a half hour of hanging around her bed, I dismissed the driver after forking over another hunk of savings. As I came back into the emergency room, we were treated to a raging drunk tied to his gurney, threatening to sue the EMS workers who brought him in. I was pleased to have been behind the procession of gurneys and EMS people when he arrived—I could give Wendy the delicious story of one of the women walking over to look at the guy and then coming back to tell her partner she'd brought him in a couple of months ago in the same condition.

"What's tomorrow going to be like?" I asked the EMS woman.

"Alcohol poisoning, busted noses, green puke everywhere," she said. "The only time it's worse is New Year's Eve."

Wendy listened to the story intently, then said, "I'm in love with my doctor. I told him, 'It's worth having a knee so swollen that it has its own zip code to be treated by you!'"

The exclamation points she was talking in were a sure clue to how scared she was and how much pain she was in. She was being cheerful, dammit! I wondered when she'd crack.

"I wish your doctor would hurry." I brushed through the curtain of her cubicle and looked around for someone who might speed this up. The X-ray, he had informed us, had confirmed her knee wasn't broken, but she'd have to have an MRI when she got back home. Then he disappeared in search of a brace and a pair of crutches. That was fifteen minutes ago.

"The woman next to me is really nice!" Wendy chatted on. "She's here with her daughter, and we commiserated about how long it all takes. I gave her my blanket because she was so cold, and they offered me cookies but I turned them down. I told them, 'I think this might be the end of my tennis career!' and we all laughed and laughed!"

It was nine thirty. I wanted to go to bed.

Oh, shit, I realized. My friends whom Wendy had stayed with were expecting company. She would have to sleep in Mimi's bed because she wouldn't be able to get up from the futon on the floor. What about Mimi? Her knees were almost as bad as Wendy's.

Her doctor, cute as a button and younger than springtime, showed up with a strappy brace and crutches. Wendy rolled up the leg of the sweatpants I'd brought, and he asked her to lift her leg. Tears sprang from her eyes as soon as she did. I excused myself and said I'd wait outside the cubicle. I saw she was grateful that I was leaving.

After some grunting from both of them, the doctor pulled the curtain back and hurried off. Wendy was sitting up, the brace lying flat under her knee.

"It doesn't fit," she sobbed. "It's one size fits all and it doesn't fit."

"Oh, honey," I said. "Remember how swollen your knee is."

"He said it was supposed to fit. He's gone off to get duct tape or something." She leaned forward as much as she could and whispered, "I gotta lose this weight, Frances. Don't ever tell anyone I said this, but I *can't* end up like Mimi! I *can't*."

I didn't tell Mimi this, of course. The next day she and I picked our way to CVS to pick up Wendy's codeine prescription and more Diet Coke. Our eyes were on every step we took, our concentration on our feet and the frozen tire grooves in the streets. It was hovering at thirty-two degrees, and we were sweating from fear and care.

Mimi came to an abrupt halt halfway down Love Lane. "This had to happen."

I looked at her to see if she was being sarcastic. She wasn't.

"Wendy needed to have this happen. I spent a lot of time talking with her last night and this morning. Every day her blog and inventory are about three things. Exercise, food, men. She needs to stop. All those things are really one thing, and she needs to step back and take stock until she understands that. She needs to learn to ask for help. This *had* to happen!"

What is truth and what is fact? Two weeks later, after blogging every day about how much she hated her knee and how big and discolored it was, Wendy learned she had arthritis and joint mice in both knees. That was a fact. The truth was harder to discern. Mimi was probably right that Wendy needed to get off her merry-go-round, but I wasn't sure Wendy understood how much she had to take the carousel's place. If she could stay in that ineffable place that is reserved for the biased observer, Wendy might pull all the bits of her—the books, Queen Victoria, the *New Yorkers*, what was on her iPod, et al— together into the confidence she had when telling a story. How we'd laughed at Teresa's on Thursday morning!

Wendy was snarking about students trickling into the bursar's off-ice to get their incomplete forms. They'd left campus in mid-January for the debutante season.

"They're *all* of them," she said, her accent making gullies and hills as she rolled across their egos, "male or female, interchangeable, 'cause they're all blonde and their names all sound like law firms. Trouble is, you call 'em by name and they have no idea who you're talkin' to. Denson Preston Nowlin maht really be a Binky, and she maht be Binkster among the Lock Jaw Set down at the Kappa Sigma house, but in the registrar's office they were all known as Tossers." Her voice dropped, and she barely moved her lips even as she lengthened the words. "As in, 'the *roo-les* are *jus'* diff'rent up here in the Big House, dahlin'. Ah'm sure you undah-*stand*' and 'Why *cain't* Ah take mah aht hist'ry exam in April?'"

"More, more," I begged. I adore the South, and Wendy knows the South from Margaret Mitchell to Bobbie Ann Mason.

"Mah favrut name of all tahm," Wendy slurred, deep in the scorn-ful heart of Appalachia, "is Candy Crystal Kane. Ah mean, did they expect her to dedicate huhself to the Daughters of the Confed'racy or become a porn stah?"

"You're kidding," Lindsay said.

"Am not. Mimi, am I kidding?"

"Unfortunately, no. And they all speak in code. 'You in on Honey Horn this year?' and counted cross stitch: 'In C-of-C Love,' thirteen stars in a St. Andrew's cross."

Mimi had seen enough homes of the good ladies—Mrs. Hus-band's-birth-name Husband's-family-name Roman numeral ("as in Mrs. Morton Cable III," Wendy translated)—of St. Alban's to be Wendy's confed'rate.

"I don't miss it at all," Mimi said as she speared another piece of French toast.

"Ah hate 'em, but ah love that they're there." Wendy shrugged.

But Wendy didn't see these things as more than facts to retell, let alone see them as her treasures. Our treasures are part of our truths.

Lindsay took two showers in her hotel room, spent the night arguing with her airline, and made it to Cincinnati and Jalen's arms as though the last couple of days had been weeks spent in the windless blue skies of the doldrums. That, too, was a fact. What was the truth? That she stood between him and a slow death from overexercise and under-eating, what the rest of us call anorexia—and he stood between her and the nicks and dings of being alone? He was her biggest project, although the married-people things they did together gave it a veneer of normalness. I wondered how disposable the rest of us were com-pared to that? I suspect more than we were to Wendy.

Mimi found a condo in Govanstown, Maryland, on a golf course. She was due to start her new job at Welch Library in mid-July, the Holly month, according to the Celtic calendar. The holly tree was her favorite tree—hardy, prickly, beautiful all year round. She thought it portentous that there were two hollies shading the entrance to her home-to-be. Their presence prompted her to throw away more stuff than she'd originally estimated, including all of her waxes and candle molds. She had an opportunity to start over and wanted to invigo-rate her Wiccan work with materials bought locally. Sleight would be behind her, and she could present some of herself as she wanted to be. Not thin, alas—or the way things were going, not thinner. But less haunted, a solitary Wicca by choice rather than command. There was an infinity to explore in her devotions. She put out feelers to the covens in the area. Jolene would be her closest friend forever, but there was more to offer back than herbs and candles.

Mimi's truth lay within her hopes and her devotion. How can you fractionate magic into facts? Any item could become holy and useful in ways the rest of us couldn't imagine.

My sweet, sad Katie kept her eyes on the pavement, sticking to facts because her truth was too tender to use. Ounces, cups, days, pounds, sales, sizes, Diet Coke, and skim milk lattes; OA meetings and OA service, making sales and contributing to the rest of the company she worked for, blogging, her cats, and her searches for the funniest YouTube postings: these were what would make her strong.

It was warming up again when I escorted Wendy to Penn Station, where a redcap took over. I was going home to a Bat Cave that would echo in its sudden emptiness. There were a thousand things to do: laundry, put dishes away, take out garbage, catch up on bills and mail, put blankets into storage, arrange my own books by my own bed, make notes. Daisy was waiting for me, napping on the couch that faces the door. She was waiting and wanting and loving ever so conditionally, but the nice thing about a dog's conditions for love is that they are mostly about being outside, playing, food, and affection. Dogs are easy to bribe into love.

The truth of my day was already written: I believed I had a thousand recoveries waiting for me. I'd used up about half of them, and I'd use up another one by the time I took Daisy out for her last pee of the night.

There is fact—the ninety-four pounds out of five hundred the Angry Fat Girls had collectively tried to lose in a year.

And there is truth—the artifacts we had made of our attempts that made our hearts bigger. We would never stop trying, but each of our bigger hearts now had room for ourselves as well as our friends. The act of solace teaches solace. We were learning to forgive ourselves because someone else had listened, understood, comforted, offered a new start whenever we were ready.

We were big with clemency as well as fat.

Lindsay posted a photo album of the loot we'd bought or exchanged and our hands fresh from manicures on Angry Fat Girlz.

Lindsay's were bright pink, Mimi's fire-engine red, Wendy's a pearly pink. Because my hands take a beating walking dogs, I went for a cleanup job and clear polish.

Two years later, I look at the photo and am surprised that Wendy's hand, although a little ungracefully sprawled, is so sensitive looking. Lindsay's is posed demurely and her wedding ring is prominent. My hand looks like a peasant's, and Mimi's is small, as fine as a dinner roll, her fingers a little stubby.

Lindsay wrote a lighthearted description of our days together.

Daisy got some extra belly rubs. Wendy, Mimi, and Lindsay all got to sleep in the Bat Cave and explore Frances's beautiful neighborhood. Frances got an excuse to clean her bathroom. A win for all involved.

In retrospect, I see in the thirteen responses to the small post the importance the blog had and how we got a kick out of it but didn't "own" the contribution we were making. One respondent gushed:

A convention. An Angry Fat Girlz convention. Can you just imagine? Would be something. All that raw power in one place. WHOOEE. I want to attend today.

But I shrugged it and the other hands in the air voting for a larger meeting off:

Actually, there wasn't much of a vibe of power, raw or otherwise. We didn't get fat because we were powerful; we got fat to hide our power. It was more of a mutual deference convention.

We all had work to do as the ice melted and the crocuses bloomed. We left it to Wendy to tell the story of her fall and long convalescence.

Mimi had responsibilities to teach and hand off. Lindsay was close to finishing her dissertation and planned to defend it in June.

And I had this book to write, the truth of my love and evolving admiration for Katie, Lindsay, Mimi, and Wendy, based on facts.

I have presented myself to you in facts only. If I'm very lucky, I am, perhaps, evolving toward a life in which the truth of me outweighs the facts.

EPILOGUE

On March 1, 2009, Lindsay, Mimi, Wendy, and I finally made the decision to cease the Angry Fat Girlz blog. Our personal lives had taken over, and we wanted to blog about our individual concerns.

Lindsay got her PhD and found a teaching job that required a move. Her time was limited, and she said in our closing statement, "The fact that I wasted so much energy agonizing over 20-ish pounds and spent so little time actually doing much about it is embarrassing. I've learned to be grateful for my body and the things I can do. I have learned that no one, besides me, gives much thought to the size of my ass."

Mimi enjoys Baltimore and her new job, but she coped with the disruption and newness by eating. She gave up Weight Watchers for a painful while, frustrated at seeing herself gain weight even as the need for knee replacement surgery grew imperative. As Asterië, she found a certain peace that she no longer found on Angry Fat Girlz, and she wanted to explore Wicca and other topics on a new blog. "We've become more balanced—and it's been a good change," she said in her adieus. Unfortunately, part of Mimi's finding balance has been an interruption (I hope it's just an interruption) in our friendship. It was too hard for her to be in communication with me while I got my abstinence together and began to lose—and blog about—serious weight.

Wendy got back together with Cal, and they are planning to move in together. Her Talbots clothes no longer fit, and with Cal in her life, she doesn't often call, although she faithfully sends me every dog cartoon that comes her way. "[Angry Fat Girlz and our readers] helped me see that we're not alone and there's more to life than a number on a scale," she concluded our nearly three years of probing so many weight-related topics and issues. On a daily basis, Wendy continues to writhe over the same things she did in this book: Cal isn't behaving the way she wants or her mother is being a pest, her boss is the Devil in Banana Republic or she's having problems with Mexican food. In the larger scheme, however, I think she's happier than she was in the year I wrote about.

Katie lost over a hundred pounds in her work with Diane, but a personal crisis dissolved her commitment to the Rooms, her food plan, and her sponsor. She gained most of it back and is currently enrolled in a medically supervised liquid fasting diet. "I had to take food out of the equation," she said. It's an extreme measure, but Katie is extreme. The doctor she sees weekly for testing has a transition program from liquid fasting to eating, and she is determined to stick to his program until she can move safely to OA or gastric bypass or a combination thereof? She hasn't committed to what will come after this course of treatment.

Last Saturday, I picked up a kelly green coin for ninety days of abstinence. It's the longest abstinence I've had in five years.

I crawled and bawled my way into the Rooms on February fifteenth after I'd blogged about how certain I was I'd be abstinent on Valentine's Day. Ah, pride. Very late on Valentine's Day, annoyed by a series of phone calls from a dog owner, I ripped my nightgown off and walked through a sleet storm to buy Sweet Cream and Cookies ice cream and a box of Oreo Cakesters. I woke the next morning in my clothes, my nightgown inside out on the bathroom floor.

"I'm so fucked up," I sobbed into Vicky's neck when she stood in the middle of the meeting and hugged me. "We're always here for you, Frances," she whispered, and pulled up a chair next to hers. A few minutes later, Patty dashed in, saw me, and beckoned me into her arms. "I'm in big trouble," I cried, and I bent down to hug her. She squeezed me hard, stepped back, and cocked her thumb and little finger in an octave, her dumb show for, "You and me. We're back together, right?" I nodded.

I hadn't cried so much or so hard in a meeting since Scott faded away from me in 2003.

A few days later, I stepped on my scale. The light in my kitchen is dim. The scale was mechanical and measured in two-pound increments. The needle went over the top weight, which I assumed to be 250 pounds but a few weeks later learned was 260. This morning I estimated I've lost thirty-nine pounds, which is also the largest weight loss I've had in five years.

Sometimes it's about the weight, but most of the time it's about what I eat. I wake each and every morning in the self-hatred of having eaten wrongly the day before. It takes a few minutes to realize I didn't. A wave of gratitude and self-respect washes over me. Because it's too hard to do it alone, abstinence means that I stay in touch with Patty. I pray to whatever God is out there.

No matter how many things may have gone wrong in the day, if I'm abstinent, I feel that I've done my job. I can be in a bear of a mood, overwhelmed with work and the idiots on the street who make my work harder, and at some point, the thought will staple itself to my brain that the next day will be better. Abstinence means I have a chance of a better day. It also puts my money in order—it costs nearly ten bucks to go out and get binge stuff. I'll be booking a trip to Prague soon from those savings. I'm more sensitive to when I'm tired; I'm more focused on my dogs, on my writing, on the DVD I'm watching, on talking to friends. I fidget and I fuss more, needing tasks like routing out dog hair or cleaning my stove.

I suffer from chronic, low-grade depression whether I'm abstinent or not, but in conjunction with drugs, when I'm abstinent, I know I can hunker down in a good book and wait it out.

Most of all, abstinence gives me hope, and hope, I learned this winter, is what operates my dreams.

In September 2008, I got an email from a college friend I had adored and looked for on all the websites she might belong to. She and a friend had recently been talking about driving up to Mount Lolo at four in the morning to see a solar eclipse at daybreak. They had invited me along and stopped to pick me up. I declined to go but gave them half a chocolate cake. The memory stirred her to look for me on Google, and she found my email address on my website. I wrote back immediately, with my phone number and a plea to give me a call.

It was as if we had spoken the day before. She giggled as she told the story of the Mount Lolo trip, and I felt ill with holding back tears she wouldn't understand. She had encapsulated me: saying no to experience because it might not fit or it might make me sweat, but handing out cake to those who went on to live while I went back to bed. We talked for most of a day and that feeling stayed with me. She had done things; I had survived things.

I stumbled around in shock from the conversation for days, hating myself. Then it occurred to me that I remembered the years we knew each other in detail and had said things like, "Oh, that was because your parents had such a great marriage." In a weird way, being side-lined had taught me to interpret what I observed. In that way, I was as necessary to her as she was to me.

Within a week of talking to her I had decided that I would, in a couple of years, move to Seattle, where she and a great many other friends and extended family live. I miss the mountains, I realized. I want Daisy to have mountains and lakes and beaches. I miss my family. I want to grow tulips and bearded iris and delphiniums, and I want a black Lab which I'll name Dahlia. I want to give a dinner party on the Spode my mother gave me when they moved to Arizona.

My dreaming mechanism awoke. There would be a million hikes in the Cascades. I would have a Christmas tree of my own. I could take sailing lessons if I wanted.

Grace boded a cycle of such reunions. On Facebook, I began to hear from people I didn't positively hate in high school and found I liked them now. And I got in touch with someone who had worked for Alix.

That was another conversation that shook me deeply. I learned how far her antics had taken her—and how low. I heard from longtime insider in the agenting world that I was a good agent, an innovator. I learned I had kept certain orders of business in the office running and that they fell apart when I was fired.

That night, Patty asked me what I felt about Alix after the conversation. "Pity," I said. I was surprised into pausing a moment. "She's self-destructive. So am I. What else can I feel if I want to get over her?"

My agent is in China at the moment. She told me she had downloaded onto Kindle the Jane Austen novel that I'm basing my own novel on. I think that means she takes me seriously and that I won't get to bask in finishing this book.

My brother Jim responded to a blog I wrote about the dream diet that he had a secret dream of his own: he wants to relay swim the English Channel in 2010. "Can I wave you off in Dover?" I emailed. My response, he said, made him cry. He went on to say no, he'd rather I welcomed him ashore in France. "In that case," I wrote back, "we'll have to rent a car and go see the battlefields in Normandy." The next day I made arrangements to start conversational French lessons.

After so many years, my capacity to dream has unstuck itself. It's abstinence that makes me able to act on my dreams.

Certain people and sugar don't mix. The measure of whether I'm one of them is whether I love sugar more than my body and my capacity to experience. The answer is obvious. Abstention gives me the chance to make the acquaintance of my body and the world. It is a rare day today. Mourning doves mew in the garden, and the sun is buttery in between the shadows of the plane trees. Cabbage roses are in perfume, and I overheard a classical violinist practicing as I walked Daisy this morning. I need lunch and a shower. Those are my facts. The truth of them is that abstinence will help me remember this day so that I can share it with you.

My desire, now, is to be neither fat nor angry anymore, and to be the girl I imagine in risky, quiet moments. I hope that anger leaves us all and that we each find our own light.

May 21, 2009

Eating Ice Cream with My Dog

READERS GUIDE

Discussion Questions:

1. What are your first memories of food?
2. At what age did you begin to gain weight?
3. At what age did you define yourself as overweight or fat?
4. At what age did you first diet? Was it your idea to restrict your food or were you put on a diet?
5. How did your parents and other authority figures talk about their and/or your weight and overeating? How did they talk about overweight people?
6. Can you estimate how many pounds you've lost in your lifetime? How many pounds you've gained in your lifetime?
7. How much influence, positive or negative, has one or more persons had over your losing weight? Why?
8. How do you and your friends talk about food, eating, weight? Do you share a common focus (e.g., wanting to lose the last five pounds or your habits of finishing your five-year-old's dinner)? If so, what sorts of strategies have you found together? If not, what is most frustrating to you about how your friends view food, eating, and weight?
9. Have you ever been embarrassed by eating or by what you've eaten?

10. Describe in detail how you think an always-thin person eats in a twenty-four-hour period.

11. Would you rather be thin or would you rather eat?

12. Consider the following emotions:
    - stress (e.g., a new job, moving, quitting smoking, boredom)
    - grief (e.g., a death, a breakup, someone moving away)
    - failure (e.g., being fired, not achieving a goal)
    - fear (e.g., starting a new career, victim of an abusive relationshiop, a sick child)

    Which of these emotions are most likely to be combined in your life? Which of them triggers memories of an earlier time in your life? Which of them is most likely to make you say, "This is not the time for me to worry about my weight or my eating"?

13. What cravings do you experience during or after a difficult day? If you fulfill your cravings, how, where, and when do you eat?

14. Fill in the blank: "If only I were the perfect weight, I would _____."
    Aside from time and money issues, could you fulfill that goal today? What have you put off in your life because of your weight?

15. Do you think you will be successful in losing and maintaining weight?

16. What three adjectives describe the best things about you?

17. What three adjectives best describe the worst things about you?

18. Describe an imaginary (or real) photo of your ideal thin self.

19. Describe an imaginary (or real) photo of your nightmare fat self.

20. Describe an imaginary (or real) photo of your actual fat self.

21. Do you think getting fat stems from the desire to eat, or the desire, conscious or unconscious, to be fat?